AGING OR ALZHEIMER'S?

AGING OR ALZHEIMER'S?

A Doctor's Personal Guide to Memory Loss, Cognitive Decline, and Dementia

Kenneth Frumkin, MD, PhD

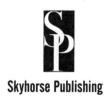

Skyhorse Publishing

Skyhorse Publishing books may be purchased in bulk at special discounts for sales promotion, corporate gifts, fundraising, or educational purposes. Special editions can also be created to specifications. For details, contact the Special Sales Department, Skyhorse Publishing, 307 West 36th Street, 11th Floor, New York, NY 10018 or info@skyhorsepublishing.com.

Skyhorse® and Skyhorse Publishing® are registered trademarks of Skyhorse Publishing, Inc.®, a Delaware corporation.

Visit our website at www.skyhorsepublishing.com.

10 9 8 7 6 5 4 3 2 1

Library of Congress Cataloging-in-Publication Data is available on file.

Cover design by David Ter-Avanesyan

ISBN: 978-1-5107-8014-9
Ebook ISBN: 978-1-5107-8015-6

Printed in the United States of America

DEDICATED TO

Bill and Ceal:
I love you. I learned more from you than I did from
over 1,200 published works.

Doctor to elderly patient: "How are you doing?"
The patient's response: "I don't know."

"If you could read my mind, love,
What a tale my thoughts could tell..."
© Gordon Lightfoot, 1970

Contents

PART IV: A GUIDEBOOK FOR THE JOURNEY

Acknowledgments

To Penny, my darling wife: Thank you for a half-century of support and the gifts of time and freedom to pursue this effort.

To Roger: You taught me what it means to care.

To Debra: You put the "pro" in pro bono, and family first in everything.

To my agent and editor, Claire Gerus: Thank you for your knowledge, your professionalism, and your friendship. Without you, I would still be writing for an audience of one.

To the librarians at the Naval Medical Center, Portsmouth, Virginia:

I asked. You always responded promptly and professionally. I could not have completed this work without you.

To Madeline Murphy: With great appreciation for your original graphic design: "Memory vs. Cognition" (Figure, Chapter 1)

To my Literary Adventure Support Group: Alan, Allen, Barbara, Charlotte, John, Nick, and Shari: Thanks for getting me to the finish line.

To Nicole Mele, formerly of Skyhorse Publishing: Thank you for seeing the value in my work. I shall always be grateful.

PART I: GETTING OLD

Introduction

Many years ago, during my medical internship, the attending physician on the neurology service shared his advice to me in words I'll never forget: "Ken, I'm going to tell you the only three words you'll need to know in order to practice neurology."

I waited, holding my breath. Somehow, I knew these words would return to haunt me.

"I'm . . . so . . . sorry," he concluded, with no hint of a smile.

Over forty years later, his words still echoing, I found myself wondering, *Where can I turn for the information I need—and the optimism I desperately crave—for my own battles with memory and aging?*

Well, what about Google? As I began searching for "dementia/memory books," 17 million results popped up. Amazon.com lists over ninety thousand books with "memory" in the title. As I perused the first few candidates on the list, I saw that most offered memory-improvement strategies aimed at students wanting to strengthen their classroom recall. Also under that umbrella were forgetful people of all ages trying to keep track of their to-do lists.

I was stunned to learn that there were currently more than ten thousand books on Alzheimer's disease. What about the National Library of Medicine? When queried in January 2023, the National Library of Medicine had cataloged 65,294 scientific papers with "Alzheimer's disease" in the title. Clearly, aging has become a huge area for investigation encompassing both potential certainties: the "now" and "the forever." Most adults are at least aware of what science and medicine advise to help them optimize their general and mental health (diet, regular medical and preventive care, exercise, moderation, social supports, etc.).

However, when seeking answers for failing memory and cognition, we have few readily available sources of unbiased information.

Instead, we are showered with opinions, hopeful predictions, statistics, pseudoscience, celebrity testimonials, and infomercials from sources both well meaning and of dubious value. With no agenda other than finding answers for myself and my family, I reviewed more than 1,200 scientific papers over nearly three years. The result is this book—a sometimes surprising, (usually) unbiased, fully referenced, and verifiable summary of the current knowledge of memory loss, cognitive aging, and dementia.

On the following pages, I will share evidence-based strategies to help you evaluate your situation and discover which solutions are available to you. Let's be honest: We all suffer from the same terminal condition—life—and there are large numbers of us who can benefit from the latest information about our aging brains. As I've learned, both as a doctor and as a private human being, knowledge is the power from which wise decisions will flow.

Why Me, as the Author of this Book?

Consider the value of an author who has dedicated years to research, analyze, and then share life-changing information about a health concern of compelling interest to both himself and his readers. Most of us have no one with whom to share our intensely personal experiences of memory loss or confusion. Yet, we all have someone we have known whose path to cognitive decline we would very much like to avoid.

I offer myself, my journey, and (informed) personal observations to fill that gap. I couldn't be more interested in this topic: now in my seventies, I find myself regularly misplacing my glasses, searching (sometimes endlessly) for a name, and deeply affected by the presence of Alzheimer's disease in persons close to me.

After years of information gathering and analysis, I firmly believe that I have consolidated on these pages what we *all* need to know about the science of aging, memory loss, and cognitive decline. My goal is to open my readers' eyes the same way I have opened mine.

The answers that matter to me, matter to you. Can we relax and slide into our "golden years," or is it time to get our affairs in order? This book examines failing memory as both a natural aging process and a possible early symptom of a devastating disease. While full-blown dementia is often apparent, there are few reliable discussions about memory fluctuations and thoughts that develop as we move from the pathway of "normal" aging to a possible berth on the "memory care" Titanic.

My research process is nearly always the same: When looking for an answer to a medical question, I search long and hard for the relevant literature, read it, analyze and synthesize what I read, and then record it in terms that I hope others will understand. For more than thirty-six years as an emergency physician, I have used the same approach to solve my individual patients' problems. I also explore, research, and publish descriptions of tested, successful therapeutic techniques, many of which my colleagues were unaware.

It won't come as a surprise when I say that the information that is readily available to the general public is—at its best—"informed opinion." Its sources are science-focused journalists attuned to press releases and other "breaking news" from the pharmaceutical industry and medical blogs. Other sources include local or national physician "experts" offering a breathless couple of minutes on the evening news.

At its worst, the information available is based on wishful thinking, hucksterism, or fraud. In contrast, the underlying science I rely on is not hidden, although many of my references are restricted to paid subscribers, or in unfamiliar online government libraries. (See my instructions for accessing those papers for free in Appendix II.) Consider this book my gift: access to data most people will not see until, possibly, it's too late.

We 70 million baby boomers have been lumped together as a statistical body throughout our entire lives. It is to these sisters and brothers that I dedicate the results of my research. As we embark on life in the later years, fellow boomers, take a deep breath. Whatever lies ahead, we can gain strength from the words, *We're all in this together.*

In the interest of "telling it like it is," I offer, in blocks like this throughout the text, my often strongly held personal opinions and observations. Although reinforced by an exhaustive literature review, these scattered "boxed" notes flow from caring for and reflecting upon tens of thousands of elderly patients and their families. They reflect my own concerns, personal and family history, hopes, fears, actions, and passions, and include anecdotes, insights, speculations, suggestions, and hopefully, some humor.

Why *This* Book, Now?

Although there are reams of books on keeping—or losing— your mental agility, there are no up-to-date single resources available to anyone planning to live beyond age sixty-four (the medical profession's definition of "elderly"). Like most people my age, I have friends and family members facing cognitive decline, plus my own "senior moments" to worry about. Being a doctor doesn't counter the dark visions of future debility that come whenever I forget a name, misplace my keys, or find myself standing in a room wondering, "Why am I here?"

Some books are a labor of love. This one is a labor of personal urgency, alternatively titled *Beat the Clock* —with me and my readers as the "intended audience." Ironically, information about memory decline continues to advance rapidly thanks to innovations across the full range of the biomedical sciences. A more urgent factor is the worldwide prevalence of dementia, with *one new case occurring every three seconds.* In fact, new information emerges so briskly that clinicians and researchers can barely keep up with it!

As I pursued my research, I learned that the most recent studies of Alzheimer's disease and its precursors were published between 2015 and 2019. These reviews all described three distinct phases of cognitive decline culminating in Alzheimer's dementia: (1) the undetectable preclinical stage, (2) mild cognitive impairment, and (3) Alzheimer's disease. In fact, the information you read in this book today is the most cutting-edge news that even your doctor may not have received! In the coming five or more years, the next summaries of the previous decade's offerings will trickle into print.

In matters of mind and memory, it's always best to have the latest data. Thus, this book is for all of us awaiting the next act in the continuing saga of aging and memory retention.

(Q): "Why all the references?" (A): "The complexity of "evidence."

Any serious researcher or writer on a subject with as much interest and concern as Alzheimer's disease will have a purpose, personal opinions, and some "evidence" (with various levels of credibility) to back up their opinions. The references I include allow others to verify or critique the information I provide. When I give my own opinion, I say so, and back it up as best I can. The little superscript numbers in the text and the pages of citations at the end are easy to ignore if there are no questions.

I chose not to cut the number of references because just telling you, the reader, "how it is" would be arrogant. In twenty-six years of education, I've been on the receiving end of far too much of that. To hide complexity by providing just one opinion would be an incorrect oversimplification. My goal is for neither you nor I to wait longer for someone else's review to address cognitive decline in ourselves or a loved one.

The most interesting data I found was new information on "subjective cognitive decline" (SCD), in chapter 2. This is now considered the *earliest* clinically identifiable set of symptoms with a risk for progression to dementia. SCD is the self-reported experience of worsening or more frequent episodes of confusion or memory loss.

When we are aware of SCD, we can benefit from earlier studies of at-risk individuals and the possibility of intervening—in some cases—before measurable decline. Right now, the specter of Alzheimer's disease is just one more thing we aging boomers fret over. We are the "target demographic" for this possible burden, haunting those of us who live long enough.

Happily, this book offers a counternarrative to the constant barrage of testimonials promoting "breakthrough" brain pills and dietary supplements. It also challenges the grim themes of TV dramas and movies that cause our children and grandchildren to view us as if *we* will soon be parented—*by them*!

"Knowledge is the antidote to fear," the wise Ralph Waldo Emerson proclaimed. It's a strength we can acquire even when other resources seem years down the road. The more current your information, the better decisions you can make. After reading this book you may have even more data than your doctor possesses about early cognitive decline!

Join me on my path to a solid understanding of the questions we seniors confront, the choices we have, and the knowledge we can safely infer from the science. Along the way, we will address the much larger and louder body of unsupported good and bad "news" vying for our attention, our hopes, and our money. Together we will explore "normal" aging of our brains, the differences between failing memory and dwindling understanding, and emerging insights into the significance of our subjective cognitive concerns.

What I share from my exhaustive review of over five hundred scientific references clarifies the biological bases, associated behavioral changes, and natural history of many seniors' number one fear, Alzheimer's disease. Topics will include risk factors for developing or progressing along the stages of cognitive decline, alternative diagnoses, the various tests and their advantages and disadvantages, plus available treatments (both longstanding and novel) and their potential for benefit. Realistic projections and practical coping suggestions for patients and families are offered.

When all is said and done, whatever the situation facing us today or tomorrow, there's one resource of strength and comfort available to us all:

The Serenity Prayer
"God, grant me the serenity to accept the things I cannot change, the courage to change the things I can, and the wisdom to know the difference."

This book brings you knowledge.
The wisdom is up to you!

Chapter 1
THE EFFECTS OF AGING ON MEMORY

You don't know what you've got 'til it's gone.

Joni Mitchell, "Big Yellow Taxi," 1970.

OK reader, you can relax. You are not alone. You have me! You have this book! Think of all the other stuff that you won't need to read (or buy!) to be ready for the age-related uncertainties facing us all. Come along for the ride as I learn about my generation's prospects for the future. Sadly, along with physical downturns, the ordinary course of cognitive aging, described in this chapter and termed "age-related cognitive decline," will inevitably complicate our maturity. Nevertheless, as my mother (and many other wise members of *her* generation) used to say, "Consider the alternative." True to the old joke, memory *is* among the first things to go, and we do sometimes forget the second, *cognition*, which is more worrisome, more dangerous, and less amenable to modification than our lost recollections.

The Nature of Memory: Categories and Definitions

We all first started worrying about memory in elementary and middle school: struggling with times tables, spelling challenges, or naming planets in order from the sun or the colors in a rainbow. But then, except for certain professions or avocations (like arts and entertainment, health care, or being a waiter in a four-star restaurant), most of us have spent the decades between secondary education and retirement without reflecting on our capability for unaided recollection. And now, memory and its failings are a near-universal concern for those of us over the age of sixty-five.

Memory involves encoding, storing, and recalling past experiences, about both the outer world and our inner processes. Different types of memories are formed and recalled by separate mechanisms found in unique areas of the brain that vary in their vulnerability to aging.[1] The various categories of memory outlined below are affected by what we will call "normal" age-related cognitive decline and neurological conditions like Alzheimer's disease. Science has identified various patterns of memory loss as indicators of specific mechanisms and locations of brain dysfunction.

Variations of Memory[2-4]

(1) *Explicit* memories from knowledge or experiences that can be consciously recalled.

(2) *Episodic* memories, which arise from combining our firsthand experiences with their context.[5] They allow us to recall personal episodes in our lives, such as: "What I did last summer," or "What I had for lunch," or "My first bite of my all-star favorite chocolate cake." Recently acquired episodic memories are more vulnerable to loss than earlier established ones.

(3) *Semantic* memories are facts and concepts about ourselves and the world. It's the system underlying our overall store of "nonspecific knowledge," such as the color of the sky or the name of your

state capital. Unlike common "tip-of-the-tongue" difficulties with recalling specific items like names and other proper nouns, impaired semantic memory leads to difficulty recalling names of common items, like "doorknob" or "toaster."

(4) *Implicit* memories come from the influence of experiences on our actions. They represent knowledge we've acquired, but cannot consciously access. Within our implicit (experiential) memories, there are three types: (a) procedural (or motor) memory enables us to unconsciously perform complex motor tasks, even though we may not be able to explain how we do them. These include riding a bicycle, playing a video game, or entering a familiar sequence of numbers on a keypad "without thinking." (b) classical conditioning results from pairing a neutral event, e.g., Pavlov's bell or a light with another stimulus (like food) that produces a natural response, such as enjoyment or salivation. Implicit memory for the association between the stimulus and response is demonstrated when the conditioned stimulus (the sound or light) begins to create the same response as the unconditioned stimulus (the food) did before the learning. (c) priming refers to influences on our behavior from recent or frequent experiences. Priming happens when particular associations are activated before you do something. If someone holds up the word *doctor*, there will be a faster recognition of the word *nurse*, than would have been given for an unrelated word.

How Long a Given Event Remains in Memory Varies Greatly

New memories pass through stages, with much forgotten along the way.

Sensory or perceptual memory is where information is first entered. New material in sensory memory stays very briefly (seconds at most) in a buffer. Unless attended to and passed on for more processing, sensory information is forgotten. Visual sensory memory is known as "iconic" memory and lasts less than a second. Auditory sensory memories ("echoic" memory) can last as long as four seconds, long enough to write down what you just heard. Some people demonstrate "eidetic" memory for details that can last a much longer time (called "photographic" memory when applied to visual stimuli).

Short-term ("working") memory includes items that are only retrievable for seconds or minutes. A short-term/working memory can be "phonological," like a phone number, or "spatial," like a route you're mentally following. We need this aspect of our memory to integrate the beginning of a sentence with its end, to mentally manipulate small bits (four "chunks") of information over several seconds, and to help us remember 5 +/- 2 items at the same time.[6]

To be retained in working memory for even that short a time, the information must often be rehearsed (like a phone number you're going to call) or manipulated (reorganized, alphabetized, or updated). Our working memories likely degrade with normal aging.[7] "Impairment" most commonly occurs when we are unable to concentrate or pay attention.

In contrast, *long-term memory* can have an almost limitless storage capacity and duration, such as "Where were you on 9/11?" The three processes central to long-term memory are encoding, storage, and retrieval. *Encoding* takes the information in the neurobiological impulses generated by our senses in response to our environment and converts it to a form that can be saved. *Storage* ("consolidation") is the very basis of learning, preserving the information absorbed and retained by the brain, commonly after sufficient repetition. *Retrieval* is the conscious, unconscious, or event-prompted process that recalls information from memory when needed.

The Effects of Aging on Memory

Typical Age-Related Changes in Memory and Cognition

In case you hadn't noticed, nothing seems to work as well after "a certain age" as it did when we were age forty or younger. Like the inevitable age-related decline in physical abilities, we experience alterations in our thinking and memory as well.[17]

Age-associated memory impairment is found in about 40% of those sixty-five or older. It is characterized by self-perceived memory loss along with a decline in objective performance on standardized memory tests compared with younger adults.[20] When subjected to the standard, brief neurological exam of reflexes, strength, eye motion, sensation, etc., healthy older people will also differ from younger cohorts.[21] Subjective concerns among this older group focus on vagueness or attentional issues, making mistakes, word and name-finding difficulties, and poor overall memory. There is also a frequency of reporting anger, frustration, or annoyance concerning memory lapses.[22]

"Am I OK for my age?" is what we begin asking ourselves. We *expect* our bodies to regress. We *know* about canes, reading glasses, and hearing aids. To what extent are our mental setbacks also a normal part of the aging process? Simply put, the difference between "normal" aging and the alternatives is the possibility of progressing to dementia.

Distinguishing what is "normal for age" from symptoms of a neurodegenerative disease is hardly new. The connection between age and memory loss has been described since 2000

BC.[8] In *The Neurology of Old Age* (1931) Macdonald Critchley, a British neurologist, was among the first of many trying to ease our concerns. He cataloged the "minor alterations in neurological signs which are typical of old age" to differentiate between "healthy old age and senility."[18] Today, such distinctions are made via the continuing development of tests and devices to detect dementia-related alterations of our brain structures and connect them with our cognitive failings.

Physiological explanations include:

(1) Regions of the brain involved in the formation and retrieval of memories often deteriorate with age, as do the levels of hormones and proteins that protect and repair brain cells and stimulate their growth.

(2) Cardiovascular disease can decrease blood flow to the brain, impairing memory and leading to possible losses in cognitive skills.

Not all memory functions are equally affected by aging. Two memory functions that remain relatively stable with increasing age include:

• Semantic memory (specific facts, like the name of the first US President), and
• Procedural memory (like riding a bicycle).

Most other memory functions are adversely affected by increasing age.[9,10] These include:

• Working memory (repeating a phone number "in your head" before dialing)
• Visuospatial skills (analyzing and mentally manipulating objects: interlocking wire puzzles or navigation)

- Processing speed (the time spent receiving, and then understanding information until you start to respond)
- Retrieval of highly specific information (names)
- Prospective memory (remembering to perform an action in the future)
- The ability to utilize new text information, while accessing and integrating prior knowledge
- Episodic memory for personal events and experiences (such as what you had for dinner) shows the greatest age-related difference.

Common Physical Infirmities That Come with Aging Can Mimic Cognitive Decline

While it is tempting to blame our senior shortcomings on an unavoidable decline in our memory, we may be ignoring the contribution of age-related physical challenges. Multiple ailments, from hardening of the arteries to hearing and vision loss, can mimic the symptoms—or hasten the onset—of neurodegenerative diseases like Alzheimer's. Along with any fading of our sensory abilities, we may find we are experiencing a clear decline in processing speed due to advancing age. This can diminish test performances on tasks that involve a timed response.

Sensory loss: For every cognitive task, we must first be able to perceive a stimulus. Only then can we process information and respond to it. Vision and hearing loss are widespread among older adults. In particular, those with hearing loss have faster rates of cognitive decline than those with normal sensory function.[12] Failing hearing and vision will often mimic memory difficulties. In the absence of well-defined visual or auditory input, the mind just fills in the gaps. When sensory failings occur, the responses can easily resemble common reactions to cognitive decline: withdrawal, depression, and fear.

Do some of us seem confused when we just can't hear the question? Did I get lost because my mind was going—or was it my sight? Sensory loss can render the standard cognitive diagnostic tests inaccurate or even invalid since they depend heavily on intact hearing and vision. (Conversely, dementia may interfere with the accurate reporting of symptoms, a necessary feature of most hearing and vision evaluations.[14])

Our auditory acuity begins to decline after age thirty, and up to 70% of subjects aged eighty or older have measurable hearing loss. With advancing age—and in settings with background noise and ambiguous speech content—speech discrimination, sound localization, and comprehension decrease. Hearing loss may be the strongest sensory barrier to cognition. While more than one sensory impairment is a statistical risk factor,[13,15] of the two, only hearing loss has been shown to affect patients' cognition and contribute to dementia.[16] Needless to say, both possibilities present risks to physical and mental health, as well as to personal safety. Remember, a fall or a car wreck will kill you a lot faster than Alzheimer's disease.

Fortunately, readily available simple evaluations and interventions can address sensory issues and potentially reduce dementia risks.[13]

Here's one way to convince Mom or Dad to finally use those hearing aids currently retired to a dresser drawer: Simply point out that whenever an older person offers an apparently unrelated answer to a question, abruptly changes the subject, or withdraws from the conversation, many people will assume that they don't understand—not that they can't hear. Ultimately, we cannot draw conclusions about ourselves or anyone else until hearing, vision, and general health have been tested and treated.

So, What Does "Normal" Mean?

The definitions of even exceedingly common terms, such as "normal" and "normal for age", often vary. What doctors, scientists, and educators mean by "normal" (at least when they are at work) is very different from common usage. For the purposes of interpreting various kinds of test results and for science in general, normal is a *mathematical* construct, not the social or behavioral one we use to judge each other. For example, the purpose of neuropsychological testing is to reliably compare a given patient's measured cognitive functions, including memory, with the average (i.e., "normal") scores of a large and appropriately matched group (similar in age, gender, race, education, etc.). In medical, statistical, and scientific matters, "normal" is used to label a subset of a larger collection of data (like test scores, lab results, or measurements) as the "most usual or common" (operationally defined as "within a specific range of the mathematical average" at the center of the typical bell-shaped random distribution of grouped data).

The "Normal Distribution"

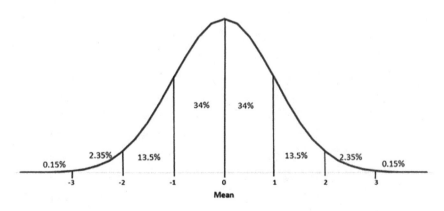

Of course, those at both ends of the bell curve are equally "abnormal"!

For some types of information (such as lab results), physicians may consider "normal" as the upper half of the curve and equate it with "desirable" and "healthy." As patients, we rarely ask what the doctor means by "normal." We just happily accept the word as an endorsement that, for now, we're OK![11]

Acceptable Levels of Cognitive Decline in Healthy Older Adults

In most research studies, regardless of the respondent's age, the "normal range" of scores (within which we all hope to fall) extends above and below the average score (the "mean") of a large number of "control" subjects who took the same test. The controls in neurocognitive testing are a group of people who are similar to the individuals being tested in age, education, gender, and other relevant factors, but *without the condition being studied.* Control-group scores establish the *standard* for normal cognitive function.

Persons being tested who do not have the condition are expected to perform similarly to the controls. Scores are statistically within the "normal range" when they fall within one "standard deviation (SD)" of the control group's mean (average). One SD includes the 34% of scores above the control-group average and the 34% below it. (See the "normal distribution" figure, above.) The highest scores on standardized tests are in young adults, which then steadily decline with age. The downward slope accelerates in old age, averaging a drop of about two standard deviations over the life span, with wide variability among individuals. When a candidate reaches two standard deviations of decline, that score aligns with the lowest 2.5% of young adults. Even so, in healthy older adults, the overall downturn in test scores is modest enough to enable them to remain independent in daily activities into the oldest age groups.[19]

Memory vs. Cognition: Looking on the Brighter Side

Many who are frustrated by memory lapses fear the worst: the onset of dementia. Here's the good news: *Failing memory is not in itself indicative of cognitive decline.* Distinguishing between pure memory loss and cognitive change requires assessing the other intellectual abilities ("domains") that combine to make up cognition. In addition to remembering, cognitive "domains" include attention, thinking, understanding, learning, solving problems, and making decisions. These are all aspects of an individual's ability to engage in activities, accomplish goals, and successfully negotiate the world.[5]

Memory "lapses" vs. memory "loss":

Our daily episodes of forgetfulness are what lead many of us to the questions that this book will answer. Authors of multiple references on memory have come to the same "logical" conclusion (admittedly, without empirical data) that:

The ability to *eventually* remember the information that we cannot immediately retrieve on demand is a *good sign*.

Although not yet officially endorsed, this is a reasonable hypothesis that I have personally taken to heart. The simple argument in favor of this hopeful opinion is: "Temporarily forgotten does not mean it's gone." The logic is: If the information sought eventually comes back, it has not been erased. Instead, you are demonstrating an age-related problem of memory retrieval. Everyone's brain cells and the pathways between them will eventually

---

age and slow. But, if we can ultimately retrieve a memory, then it (and the connections to it) has not been obliterated or displaced by the abnormal proteins that define Alzheimer's disease (AD).

Many memory lapses are *not* considered warning signs of dementia.[23,24] These include:

- Sometimes forgetting where you left items you use regularly, like glasses or keys, but you can retrace steps and locate them again.
- Forgetting names of acquaintances or replacing one memory with a similar one, e.g., the very common occurrence of running through several relatives' names before landing on the intended one.
- Occasionally getting confused about the day of the week, missing an appointment, or walking into a room and wondering why you entered, but remembering later.
- Becoming easily distracted or having trouble recalling what you've just read, or the details of a conversation.
- Sometimes having trouble in finding the right word, or not quite able to retrieve information on the tip of your tongue. It will, happily, reappear later during another conversation.
- Occasional math errors.
- The ability to recall and describe instances of forgetfulness.
- Having to pause to remember directions, but not getting lost in familiar places.

- Waning tolerances: sometimes becoming weary of work, family, and social obligations or preferring to do something in a certain way and becoming irritated when your routine is disrupted.
- Occasionally making questionable decisions, but overall sound judgment and decision-making ability rule the day.

There may be newer types of memory loss still to be investigated and characterized. For example, (1) "Password/PIN amnesia" and (2) "What the heck did I order from Amazon two days ago?" Good news! After numerous "interviews" with much younger folks, I realized that the phenomenon of "What did I order?" is triggered when the package appears! This seems neither an age-related memory issue nor a sign of dementia.

Definitions of "Normal for Age" Will Inevitably Change

We must, alas, be aware that the pedestal of "normal for age" upon which we all hope we stand is being whittled away by medical progress. New tools, from latest-generation scanners to AI (artificial intelligence), to genetic and bio-diagnostic tests, may shine an unwelcome light on our inner idiosyncrasies even before we develop symptoms.[25] It will become harder to cling to "normal for age" status when every year uncovers more ways to spot ominous abnormalities in our brains, biofluids, gene sequences, and in one-on-one neuropsychological testing.

Maintaining the comfort of "normal" will require that these new and depressing alternative explanations have been ruled out. Since definitive tests (see chapter 4) can be invasive, expensive, and unavailable to many, uncertainties will persist. As we identify more abnormalities to exclude and develop the means to do so, what is "normal for age" will undoubtedly change.

In addition, the various labels commonly applied to memory loss also lack consistent definitions. Confusion is such that, in its 2015 monograph on cognitive aging, the National Academy of Medicine (the health branch of the US National Academy of Sciences) specifically avoided the term *normal aging*.[5] Common terms like *senior moments* are *not* medical diagnoses and are without assigned scientific meaning. This is equally true for "mild memory loss associated with aging," which is supposedly improved by Prevagen®. This heavily marketed dietary supplement made from transmogrified jellyfish proteins appears on a near-continuous nightly cycle in TV commercials.[26] (Prevagen® is fully discussed in chapter 5.)

And, if you're wondering about normal memory loss vs. dementia, you can take the following quiz from AARP: https://www.aarp.org/health/brain-health/info-2015/normal-memory-loss-vs-dementia-quiz.html#quest1.

Speaking of Quizzes:

Attention Baby Boomers: If you can remember the name of this magazine *Cover Boy*, the name of the magazine, and the caption that goes with his picture, your long-term memory *may be OK*. See *Cover Boy* in the Glossary (Appendix I) for the answer.

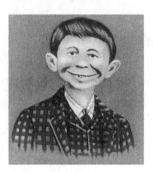

Cognitive Decline is Memory Loss's "Evil Twin"

For many in their sixties and older, memory and cognition are the two sides of a coin stolen from them by Father Time. The various forms of memory loss have been described earlier, and now you will learn more about "cognition."

Think of cognition as the difference between "remembering" and "knowing." With aging, memory difficulties are more common, more "normal," and appear earlier than any of the more consequential cognitive changes. As to the "evil twin"—when we develop cognitive failures, they may be incorrectly perceived as worsening memory, masking or delaying our recognition of cognitive decline's more serious threats to our safety and independence. It's one thing to forget why you went to the mall (memory) and quite another to be unable to find your way home.

A second example is illustrated in the Figure below. In this case, we can observe the difference between *forgetting* where you put your keys and *knowing* how to unlock a door.

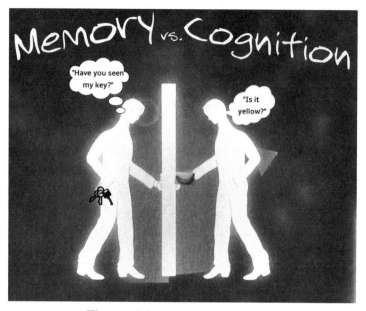

Figure: Memory vs. Cognition

Age-Related Cognitive Decline (ARCD)

Age-related cognitive decline (ARCD) is the preferred term commonly substituted for phrases such as "normal, normal for age, normal cognitive decline with aging, age-related memory loss, senior moments," etc. Terms used will still vary a bit, based on the context (i.e., the details of the study and the intended audience).

The word *cognitive* is the key, encompassing more domains than just memory. Most of the time, your doctor will assign you to that category (ARCD) based on your history, the clinical impression you present, and a "normal" score on one of the brief primary-care–based, in-office tests like the Mini-Mental Status Exam (MMSE). Reassurance and follow-up are, for now, the most common responses to achieving membership in the ARCD category. (See chapter 2.)

Specific Cognitive Changes With ARCD[27,28]

The patterns of cognitive change that occur with ARCD tend to start after age sixty.

Six cognitive domains can be variously affected by aging. They are memory, language, attention, learning, executive functions, and visuospatial abilities.

Memory: Within the cognitive domain of memory there are multiple common recall failures that can occur with "normal" aging and therefore be seen early and frequently with ARCD.

(1) Source memory (i.e., accurately knowing the origin of the information) declines with age, as does the level of detail of recalled *episodic memories* of personal experiences.

(2) Prospective memory, specifically remembering to perform an intended action in the future (e.g., taking medication after breakfast), also declines with age.

(3) Working memory and encoding: Tests that require subjects to exceed the normal memory storage capacity of six to seven items are more difficult for older adults. Working memory—the small amount of information that can be held and used to execute cognitive tasks—also requires being able to manipulate new information. This process declines with age.

(4) Retrieval of information may require more cueing or a specific format to remain stable in advanced-age groups.

Language: Speech production (verbal fluency, verbal retrieval, and some naming tasks) also drops off with age. When compared with young adults, seniors were less verbose, more repetitive, and less specific in word choice in spontaneous speech.

Attention: Complex tasks are most affected by age-related changes in attention. "Selective attention" is the ability to focus on specific information in an environment while simultaneously ignoring irrelevant information. "Divided attention" is the ability to focus on multiple tasks simultaneously, such as walking on an obstacle course and answering questions.

Learning and the Retrieval of Learned Material: New learning declines with aging and becomes more difficult for older adults if the test requires manipulating new information in one's working memory. Another challenge, "divided attention," arises if subjects must split their attention among multiple activities at the same time they're learning new information.

Executive Cognitive Functions: These are decision-making, problem-solving, reasoning, processing speed, the planning and sequencing of responses, and multitasking. All get worse with advancing age.

Visuoperceptual Judgment: The ability to organize and interpret what is seen, and give it meaning, diminishes with age, along with the ability to perceive spatial orientation and copy a complex design. On free-drawing tasks, pictures drawn by older adults become more simplified and less detailed.

Overall Performance: Performance on tests that are novel, complex, or timed will steadily decline. These include standard IQ measurements, scores on tests that require inhibiting some responses but not others, and those involving an ability to distinguish between relevant and irrelevant information.

Concept formation, abstraction, and mental flexibility also fade, especially after seventy.

Some Cognitive Abilities May Remain Stable With "Normal Aging"

(1) Memory: Some aspects of memory are preserved or can even *improve* with age, including delayed recall, general knowledge, vocabulary, recognition, historical memories for public events; autobiographical (episodic) memory; immediate or "sensory memory"; procedural memories, such as remembering how to play the piano or ride a bike; and retaining newly learned information.

(2) Attention: Simple tasks such as digit span (the ability to repeat a series of digits of increasing length) are maintained in normal subjects up to age eighty.

(3) Speech and language remain largely intact. Vocabulary, verbal reasoning, and comprehension in normal conversation all remain into advanced age.

(4) Visual recognition of objects, shapes, gestures, and conventional signs remains stable into advanced age, and a person's ability to copy a simple figure is not affected.

The Differences Between Memory and Cognition are Worth Emphasizing

Both will worsen with age. "Normal" age-related loss of memory (the storage and recall of past experiences) is a quantitative change, generally paralleling the many other measurable changes that come with time. On the other hand, what we recognize as "cognition" is the integration within the brain of distinct intellectual functions involved in attention, thinking, understanding, learning, problem-solving, and decision-making.[29] More than memory and recall, cognitive functions are "fundamental to an individual's ability to engage in activities, accomplish goals, and successfully negotiate the world."[5]

Once significant subjective or objective decline develops within a *cognitive domain*, the focus needs to broaden from the neural connections involved in memory and forgetting to the clinical and biological stages that underlie the cognitive decline of Alzheimer's disease. When cognitively normal older adults underwent repeated neuropsychiatric testing over six years, declines in verbal and working memory were not "age-related." Instead, they were attributable to the identified presence of unrecognized amyloid (preclinical AD).[30]

While the symptoms of "cognitive decline" can initially be mild, or even completely subjective,[29] they signify a detectable deterioration of cognition with age. Going beyond failing memory—they can foretell the evolution from normal aging to dementia.

You *will* have *memory* failings as you get older. *Cognitive decline*, however, is far from inevitable, and nowhere near as funny as your kids and grandkids might think (or you might pretend). Even if you are the only one who notices, check it out! (See chapter 3.)

Remember: *Dementia is diagnosed when cumulative failures of both memory and cognition interfere with everyday activities.*

PART II: THE UNEVEN PATH TO DEMENTIA

Chapter 2
SUBJECTIVE COGNITIVE DECLINE (SCD)

What comes after "normal" age-related cognitive decline? Most of the time, nothing more than an increasing dependence on Post-it® notes, and the continued frustrations of wondering, again, why you're in the closet, or where you left your keys. But if the potential for progression is in your future, you will be the first to know! The most recently added proposed stage in cognitive deterioration is diagnosed by the answer to a simple question that you ask yourself. Save your time and money, and skip the embarrassing clock drawing, object-naming, and "Where are we?" questions.

Subjective cognitive decline (SCD) is the most recently identified stage of dementia and, by definition, the earliest one we can discover ourselves. "New" stages of any disease (even one identified over a century ago) arise upon the recognition, first by patients, then by clinicians, of symptomatic and behavioral patterns that have proven to predict the same outcome.

Defined in 2014 by a working group of international researchers and clinicians,[31,32] SCD is the "*self-reported* experience of worsening or more frequent confusion or memory loss within the previous 12 months."[33]

SCD is identified by two primary characteristics: (1) Any deterioration (failing memory or progressive confusion) is, from the individual's perspective, unrelated to an acute event. An observation of decline by others is not required. (2) Performance on standardized cognitive tests remains normal.

The importance of subjective concerns has varied widely over decades, influenced by the lists of "Stages of Alzheimer's disease" offered up by various researchers and later adopted by international experts in "working groups." Early observers proposed that a patient's self-perception of "the forgetfulness phase" was the first stage of AD.[34,35]

"Subjective decline" remains in clinical use as Stage 2 of Reisberg's Global Deterioration Scale (GDS), a seven-level description of dementia progression. That stage includes "subjective complaints *without* objective change." For example, the patient complains: "I can't remember anything, Doc, not even what I had for breakfast," but then aces an in-office memory test like those in the Mini-Mental Status Exam.[35-37]

Subjective concerns were initially considered as a criterion for mild cognitive impairment, the stage that immediately precedes AD.[38,39] Eventually, the anatomical confirmation of SCD as a distinct AD Stage 2 came when 40% of individuals who consulted memory clinics with subjective complaints were found to have positive amyloid biomarkers. This added value and focus to an SCD diagnosis as a time for early intervention and risk factor modification.[40]

This chapter is the one most important to me and readers like me: those beginning to forget more *and* wondering what might be coming next. The drive to seek the information within this book arose when I came upon the most recent medical literature identifying SCD and its role in overtaking "normal" aging. SCD is not yet widely studied, mainly because it was recognized *after* the most recent batch of authoritative ten-year publications about Alzheimer's disease published between 2015 and 2019.

SCD will likely be featured more prominently when multi-authored "state-of-the-art" updates are rewritten a decade from now. I chose not to wait, for both my benefit and for yours. The evolving information described here validates our natural resistance when a doctor's reassurance of "normal for your age" fails to match our own assessments.

More Than Memory Loss

"Memory" involves recalling past experiences. "Cognition" is our ability to analyze and synthesize facts or develop new ideas using language, planning, and attention in addition to memory. It is when *both* memory and cognition decline, leading to the inability to perform daily activities, that defines the stage known as "dementia."

Most SCD evaluations are triggered by the subjective memory concerns of up to half of older adults. Any deterioration in cognitive domains as well as memory should be included when assessing SCD. This makes memory issues highly sensitive, but not specific enough to reliably detect preclinical AD in the form of SCD.[41,42]

In addition to memory (at 66.9 %), the cognitive domains most affected in SCD patients include attention (54.6%), motor (52.9%), executive (functioning 39.7%), and language domains (31.5%). In all these domains, SCD prevalence increased with age and was strongly associated with symptoms of depression and, to a lesser extent, with emotionality.[42]

SCD: Its Role in the Study and Management of Dementia

So, is SCD the doorway to Alzheimer's disease, or just another concern of the "worried well"? First and foremost, the driving force to understand SCD was the generation of baby boomers. We just kept on complaining about our memory issues and seeking answers from our health-care systems. After having joined the "worried well" and suffering the same "senior moments" we saw in our parents and grandparents, we fretted that even worse could be on its way! To further stoke our fears, there was no name for this process, and no research findings to answer our lingering questions. (This despite our repeated and reassuring demonstrations to our doctors that we could draw a clock *and* remember three items five minutes after hearing their names).

It makes sense to be concerned! Finding those at the earliest stage of decline is the best way to select populations for targeted dementia research and prevention trials.[31] It's not as if doctors aren't aware of the frequency of our unverifiable cognitive complaints. According to Doctors Budson and Solomon in their 2022 textbook, *Memory Loss, Alzheimer's Disease and Dementia*: "Some patients present to our clinic certain that their memory has declined over time, yet when we give them detailed neuropsychological testing they perform normally, even when we take into account their age and education."[43]

Fortunately for your doctors, there is an official—and billable—ICD-10 code for the diagnosis of "no diagnosis" (The code is z71.1—"person with a feared complaint in whom no diagnosis is made").[44] SCD patients are otherwise (cognitively) healthy. By definition, they do not perform worse on standard psychometric test batteries than those without memory complaints.[45]

Unfortunately, as with so many of our interactions with the health-care system (and commerce in general) the seller gets paid, our lives move forward, and (as continued below) what progress is made stays largely behind the scenes.

Establishing SCD as a "New Stage" of Alzheimer's Disease

To avoid confusing apples and oranges, reliable criteria are required to identify SCD patients and differentiate them from those with similar subjective concerns—but without the risk of progression to AD. Objective diagnostic criteria are always the best way to combine patients into groups for study and potential treatment. However, it has not been clear as to how to objectively evaluate a condition that presents subjective complaints but lacks abnormalities upon neuropsychological testing.

Attention to this dilemma began in the medical literature at the end of the last decade. SCD, although currently studied by increasing numbers of researchers, is still an "unofficial" diagnostic category, with low levels of knowledge, recognition, and acceptance in the medical community. Until they can read the upcoming decade's reviews, your doctors may choose to see you and your distress over subjective cognitive symptoms as yet another member of the "worried well" genre, not as a person undergoing the second stage in the development of Alzheimer's disease."

Because it is so new, information on SCD is hard to find. It is not yet listed in the *International Classification of Diseases* (ICD),[46,32] which assigns codes to specific diagnoses, the *American Psychiatric Association Manual*,[32] relevant textbooks published before 2022,[47,48] or the Research Framework of the National Institute on Aging and Alzheimer's Association (NIA-AA).[49] For other conditions, ICD and other codes are the way to track statistics like hospitalizations, disease frequency, outcomes, and billing.

> SCD might get a lot more love if doctors could bill under a specific diagnosis.

It appears that comparatively little work on SCD is ongoing. As recently as 2020, memory researchers still referred to SCD as "controversial," or "proposed."[50] At the end of 2022 there were just 601 works with "subjective cognitive decline" in the title in the entire National Library of Medicine database, with the first published in 2014. In comparison, there were over thirty-two thousand references with titles including "Alzheimer's disease" published during the same period.

OK, Boomers—Maybe We're All Just the "Worried Well"?

Alas, "SCD deniers" do tend to label us that way. Fortunately, not every physician finds this an appropriate label. One doctor wrote, "Calling patients the 'Worried Well' is disrespectful and doctor-centered . . . if a doctor is in a negative mindset, they are less likely to take the opportunity . . . to foster health promotion and build relationships."[51]

Officially recognized or not, SCD resembles what many seniors experience or recognize in others, and what every educational curriculum, textbook, or symposium addressing cognitive loss has either been unaware of or has chosen to ignore. Our self-perceived declines in cognitive capacity, the same concerns that caused me to write this book and brought many of you to read it, have yet to find resonance with the experts to whom we take our growing concerns.

Might we benefit from more than a patronizing dose of reassurance, dispensed by a "specialist" stranger in a white coat? One nationally recognized expert (whom I traveled nine hundred miles to see) put it as courteously to me as I have ever heard it said to an anxious patient: "At this time, nobody would diagnose you with an aphasia. On the other hand, it is also true that people with a lot of insight and who are functioning at a very high level can detect changes in themselves way before any kind of test that we have can pick that up."

This left me with a non-medical question: "Are left-handed compliments the new reassurance?" Flying home from that appointment, I found myself a freshly reassured member of the worried well, recently retired and looking towards the next stage of my life, blessed with financial security, a loving family, education, good insurance, and relatively easy access to leading experts. And, of course, I had a normal twenty-minute office neurological exam.

But then . . . I came across a body of work describing SCD, a formerly unreviewed entity populated with people like me, and having an annual rate of conversion to the next stage of cognitive decline (MCI) of 7% per year.[35]

Now, much less reassured but empowered by a plausible new diagnosis to investigate, I vowed to continue my search of medical literature to pass on to the millions of other "worried well" out there.

Who Has Subjective Cognitive Symptoms?

Prevalence: When asked, 50–80% of individuals aged seventy and older who scored within normal ranges on cognitive tests reported some form of self-perceived decline in cognitive functioning.[32,83]

In almost eight thousand British adults fifty years and over, the prevalence of any subjective cognitive complaint was 46.5%. This increased with age and was more common in women.[84] Twenty-five to forty percent of those seeking help for cognitive decline in two memory clinics in Europe met the criteria for SCD.[32]

In one "dementia-free adult population," 53% of nearly nine thousand participants forty to seventy-nine years old had "subjective cognitive symptoms."[85] Using the CDC's self-definition question: *During the past 12 months, have you experienced confusion or memory loss that is happening more often or is getting worse?*[29,33] the overall prevalence of SCD among adults over forty-five is roughly 11%, and is nearly the same in men and women.[29]

Social Demographics: Among racial and ethnic groups, 11% of Caucasians reported SCD, compared to 13% of African Americans, 11% of Hispanics, and 7% of Asians and Pacific Islanders.[29] SCD with lowered performance in memory and verbal fluency tasks was present in 18.5% of dementia-free community-dwelling older adults and was associated with professional activity, quality of life, neuroticism, and current depression.[42,86]

These may seem like small differences, but disparities in the prevalence of even one to two per hundred older folks is a significant public health issue when considering the increasing millions of elderly here and around the world.

Risk Factors for Developing SCD

Advancing age is the most powerful overall predictor of risk for the development of AD or any of its precursors.[87]

Living alone: On average, 29% of adults with SCD live alone. Of those aged forty-five to sixty-four, 25% with SCD live alone compared to 36% of those sixty-five and older. Thirty percent of women with SCD live alone compared to 28% of men. Among racial/ethnic groups with SCD, 30% of

Caucasians live alone compared to 35% of African Americans, 18% of Hispanics, and 15% of Asians and Pacific Islanders.[29]

Education: A lower prevalence of SCD is reported in adults with more years of formal education. [88]

History of traumatic brain injury (TBI): Defined as altered brain function caused by blunt or penetrating injury to the head, a history of TBI is often present in patients with SCD. While the mechanisms by which TBI leads to cognitive decline have yet to be fully elucidated, the more severe the head injury, the worse the cognitive consequences.[89]

Being a caregiver: A CDC report found that one in eight adult unpaid caregivers for a family member or friend with a health condition or disability experienced more frequent confusion or memory loss over the preceding year.[90]

Other risks: In a study of 1,165 participants without objective cognitive impairment and showing an overall SCD prevalence of 42%, the frequency of SCD gradually rose as the number of eight identified risk factors increased. Four factors (older age, thyroid diseases, minimal anxiety symptoms, and daytime dysfunction) were associated with *both* SCD and its severity, while the others (female sex, anemia, lack of physical exercise, and living alone) were linked with either SCD *or* its severity.[91]

Diagnosing SCD

It's a significant decision to label an individual with isolated subjective complaints as having SCD (potentially, "early Alzheimer's"). Doing so indicates the possibility of *further* cognitive decline. Therefore, to diagnose SCD one needs to take the following steps:

(1) Verify the presence of clinical diagnostic features of SCD patients that distinguish them from their

peers with "normal" age-related cognitive decline (ARCD),

(2) Exclude the possibility of MCI with negative cognitive testing results.

(3) The effect of studies that confirmed the distinctions among ARCD, SCD, and MCI was the addition of SCD (renamed "subjective cognitive impairment") to the stages of cognitive decline in the elderly. The downhill path is now described as going from "normal for age" to "subjective decline," to "mild cognitive impairment," to "dementia."[52]

The "SCD Question"

In numerous research studies by the US Centers for Disease Control and Prevention (CDC) and others, SCD patients *without* MCI or other explanations for their concerns have been identified for study by their affirmative answer to what can be called the "$64,000 SCD Question":

During the past 12 months, have you experienced confusion or memory loss that is happening more often or is getting worse?[29,33]

Although proven valuable for studies and surveys, those with positive answers to this question are a heterogeneous group with preclinical AD in 20–25%, subthreshold psychiatric symptoms in more than a third, and the rest without evidence of either.[53]

"SCD-Plus" Diagnostic Criteria

The following is a list of clinical features suggestive of a neurodegenerative disorder. Their presence can separate SCD from both age-related cognitive decline (ARCD) and the "worried well."[29,31,32,53-57]

SCD-plus clinical features include:

(1) Subjective decline in memory, regardless of function in other cognitive domains;
(2) Onset within the past five years;
(3) Onset at age sixty or older. (Those younger than sixty are more likely to have other or potentially reversible causes of SCD, like depression);
(4) "Concerns/Worry": Those who worry significantly along with their perceived decline are at increased risk of objective decline or dementia in the future;
(5) Persistence of SCD longer than six months;
(6) Seeking medical help;
(7) Confirmation of cognitive decline by an observer.

In the absence of alternative explanations or positive neurocognitive testing, the presence of SCD-plus criteria both confirms the diagnosis of SCD and *increases* the possibility of having positive AD biomarkers.[58]

An SCD summary score (SCD-I) that correlates with the presence of AD biomarkers can be generated from a structured interview. It is calculated by adding the number of SCD-plus features (see previous paragraph) present to the number of cognitive domains affected.[56]

Diagnostic Questionnaires

These use both self-reports and observations by caretakers or others when assessing for SCD. The SCD score of *subjective cognitive function*, a self-report mailout test for cognitive deterioration, is calculated from yes-or-no answers to six questions with one point for every yes.[57,59]

(1) "Do you have more trouble than usual remembering recent events?"
(2) "Do you have more trouble than usual remembering a short list of items, such as a shopping list?"
(3) "Do you have trouble remembering things from one second to the next?"
(4) "Do you have any difficulty in understanding things or following spoken instructions?"
(5) "Do you have more trouble than usual following a group conversation or a plot in a TV program due to your memory?"
(6) "Do you have trouble finding your way around familiar streets?"

Two scores at different times were averaged and classified as good (0), moderate (0.5–2.5), and poor (3–6 points). Validation came from scoring subjects in two studies following more than seventy-seven thousand health professionals over decades. Over time and repeated surveys, low SCD scores were associated with fewer known risk factors for SCD and fewer subsequent cases of dementia.[59,60]

You could just go ahead and try it! But recognize that these six simple questions have the potential to deconstruct your life! Remember, the SCD score is a research tool that calculates the odds of SCD in a group. Such scores cannot make predictions for individuals. Talk to your doctor before taking any such tests.

Questionnaires: self-report vs. informants. The accuracy and relative value of the two methods vary throughout early AD.[61] Self-reports may be most meaningful at the earliest (pre-clinical) stage. For concerned but cognitively normal subjects, informant reports tend to correlate better with progressive objective findings,[57] while some combinations of self-and-informant reports have been better than either alone.[62,63]

Predicting SCD

Not surprisingly, new and more specific tests to expose *tendencies* towards developing SCD—even before subjective decline—are still in development.[35]

Proving the Negative: ("It's not MCI or dementia!")

By definition, self-perception of cognitive decline (SCD) does not require confirmation by external observation.[31] The second requirement for a diagnosis of SCD is normal objective neuro-cognitive testing to rule out MCI and dementia. Unfortunately, the short, in-office screening tests like the MMSE or Montreal Cognitive Assessment are inadequate, both for identifying MCI and for differentiating it from SCD. The best recommendations to differentiate MCI from SCD are normal scores on comprehensive tests for which age, sex, and education-adjusted normative data are available.[32]

Be prepared—it will be a long day of testing! Scores vary widely, even among cognitively normal adults.[19] Up to 30% of adults over sixty-five who tested "normal" still met clinical criteria for SCD[64] and positive answers (MCI) may come too late, missing a window for potential research or intervention.

Do I Have SCD?

If you are ready to face your fears, you can ask yourself the "SCD Question":

During the past 12 months, have you experienced confusion or memory loss that is happening more often or is getting worse?

"The Question" has been used by the CDC for large surveys and other studies, and served as the basis for their 2019 publication *Subjective Cognitive Decline—A Public Health Issue* (https://www.cdc.gov/aging/data/subjective-cognitive-decline-brief.html) Remember, among those with positive answers, uncertainty will continue. Preclinical AD was found in only 20–25%[53] and there is no way to know at the time you answer the question, into which group you will fall!

If your answer to the SCD Question is "Yes," and, after consulting with your doctor, *you must know,* a next step would be biomarker testing (see the discussion that follows).

Brain and Body Fluid Biomarkers in SCD

What are Biomarkers?

Biomarkers (discussed here, and more fully in chapter 4) identify the presence of the proteins that define AD which, for over half a century, could only be diagnosed during an autopsy.[65] The presence of biomarkers was used to validate a number of the tests and questionnaires used to identify SCD.[32,53,56,57,66,67] Finding markers in patients meeting other criteria for SCD separated that new diagnosis from asymptomatic preclinical states.[50] It also displaced MCI (with its requirement for positive neurocognitive tests) as AD's first diagnosed stage. In cognitively unimpaired individuals over age sixty, the larger the brain biomarker load, the greater the severity of subjective cognitive concerns.[32]

Biomarker prevalence in those with SCD: Spinal fluid AD biomarkers were more common in those with subjective complaints than in control subjects (52% vs. 31%).[54] Those with SCD showed more brain atrophy;[32,68-70] reduced cerebral metabolic activity,[71] and positive markers for amyloidosis and neurodegeneration.[54,55] In individuals with SCD seeking medical help, the number with at least one biomarker present (amyloid or tau) increased with age and ranged from lows of approximately 7–10% to 40–76%.[32,66]

Should I Get Biomarker Tests If I Think I Have SCD?

For better or for worse, those of us with subjective concerns are potentially just one biomarker test away from a near-certain diagnosis of underlying Alzheimer's disease.

Biomarkers, cautions and caveats: There is great variability and major limitations when researching the associations between biomarkers of Alzheimer's disease and SCD.[32] Some studies fail to demonstrate any relationship at all between the presence of biomarkers and subjective memory complaints in the "healthy elderly."[54]

With newer and more sensitive techniques, neuropathological changes are being found in a high proportion of adults over sixty who show "no impairment" in cognition, mood, or behavior (i.e., preclinical).[30] Conversely, subjective memory complaints are found in the vast majority of adults over sixty, even though only a small proportion of them are biomarker-positive (<30% at that age).[58]

Here's the good news: *The presence of biomarkers does not guarantee progression to AD!* In one study of 151 SCD patients undergoing multiple biomarker assessments: 25% had preclinical AD (biomarker positive), 38% had psychiatric symptoms, while the largest group of participants (43%) did not have evidence of either. Other limitations of the association between AD bio-markers and SCD include: (1) Just a few reports, with various settings and definitions, have examined this association. (2) No long-term studies have followed biomarkers in initially unim-paired individuals through subsequent objective decline. (3) Studies focusing on markers other than amyloid and tau pro-teins are needed, as these two markers do not account for SCD in other neurodegenerative diseases.[31]

Those previously identified (blown off?) as the "worried well" will get a lot more to worry about from the science of biomarkers. A negative test would be very reassuring. On the other hand, a positive test would mean going from expert reassurances of "Relax, it's all in your head" to "It is all in my head!!"

An argument against testing: Look, the odds are in your favor. The vast majority of individuals with SCD do not progress to dementia but rather remain cognitively normal.[72] Plus, there is insufficient data to establish whether, *for any individual,* biomarkers can predict the progression of cognitive decline.[32]

We need to keep reminding ourselves: It is statistically impossible to confidently predict the outcome for any one patient from their inclusion in a group with less than a 100% likelihood of the result in question. Put another way, a positive answer gives one a 100% probability of worrying about a 25% possibility.

Maybe test, go ahead, and roll the dice! Biomarker positivity is newly described in SCD. A positive test at such an early stage of AD would offer the maximum amount of time to plan for a now-uncertain future. False positive biomarker tests are rare, so the predictive value of a negative test is high. *The optimum clinical benefit of testing for SCD is to reassure individuals with normal biomarkers.*[72] Decades of subsequent worry can be prevented. Doctors writing on this subject tend to wimp out on the question of testing by advising that "clinical decisions for those with SCD actively seeking medical help should be *tailored to their individual needs.*"[32]

You may well feel that there is something wrong before any tests turn abnormal—or before your doctors discuss the possibility that your symptoms could be more than "old age." Increasing recognition and respect for the value of "individual needs" means increasing respect for the patient. (And maybe less time minimizing our concerns until the day we can no longer draw that stupid clock!)

What Are the Risks and Benefits of an Early Presumptive Diagnosis of SCD?[73]

Risks: Emotional distress, depression, anxiety, impaired medication adherence, and overall reduced quality of life can occur. As patients age with this diagnosis, it can be difficult to avoid stressing out over every inevitable "senior moment." Some might withdraw by limiting driving, social contact, and financial responsibilities to avoid making mistakes. SCD patients may consume unnecessary and potentially harmful over-the-counter regimens or seek phony procedures promoted to stimulate memory.

Benefits: Awareness of SCD provides an opportunity to address the harmful anxiety or depression that often accompanies it. An evaluation of potential causes of SCD could uncover a reversible condition.

Genetic Markers in SCD (APOE4)

Other than a proliferation of amyloid and tau proteins, there is no biological contributor to Alzheimer's disease better supported by multiple sources of evidence than the E4 variant of the apolipoprotein E (APOE) gene, APOE4. Gene sequencing is not a "biomarker." Biomarkers reveal the current presence of abnormal brain proteins that can eventually generate interference with memory, cognition, and function—AD. The presence of an Alzheimer's-related gene sequence is a "risk factor" for AD. It is not a cause, but an inherited tendency to develop AD *under certain circumstances.* (See chapter 4.)

Individuals with SCD:

- have a greater frequency of expression of APOE4, especially those with positive biomarkers.[54] ("Expression" occurs when a gene is induced to manufacture its associated protein.)
- demonstrate significant anatomic changes in multiple brain locations compared to SCD individuals without the gene.[74]

Carriers of the APOE4 gene with self-reported cognitive concerns experience cognitive decline more rapidly than non-carriers.[75,76] Those cognitively intact but above the age of seventy have a greater chance of developing SCD[77], and carriers with SCD or the SCD-plus criterion of age $\geq$ 60 have increases in multiple AD biomarkers.[53,66,69,78-82]

What Else Could It Be?

Not all subjective memory complaints can be attributed to preclinical Alzheimer's disease. Other items in the differential diagnosis include normal aging, personality traits, and psychiatric disorders and their treatments. [54] At younger ages, the likelihood of SCD due to causes other than AD increases.[92] Below age sixty, the likelihood of a medical condition causing future cognitive decline and dementia is lower than in the over-sixty group. The chance is higher that SCD in the younger group is from potentially reversible causes (e.g., depression).[32]

Psychological States and Neuropsychiatric Conditions[54,93]

Anxiety: In cognitively unimpaired seventy-year-olds, symptoms of SCD are more often associated with anxiety traits than with amyloid pathology. Thus, it is necessary to consider anxiety symptoms prior to assessing for AD and SCD.[94] This is particularly important because anxiety can be treated.

Other psychological conditions include: psychosomatic disorders (i.e., physical symptoms prompted by psychological factors or conflict, without associated objective findings); "sensitive self-monitoring" (a personality trait in which persons very concerned with how they present themselves in public monitor and adjust their behaviors to accommodate social situations); neuroticism and fears of dementia can trigger patient concerns about cognitive decline or strongly amplify the experience of normal age-related changes.[32]

"Worried well" is a label applied to those concerned that they may have dementia, but are "neurologically normal relative to others in their demographic upon examination and testing."[95] This group is more likely to have personal relationships with dementia patients, like relatives with dementia (particularly known APOE4 carriers). They often suffer from heightened vigilance about their perceived cognitive failings and have excessive concerns about their level of function. They continue to worry and may even display higher rates of cognitive deterioration than less concerned peers.[32,83,96] Some psychiatrists (the medical specialty that gets paid to listen, and has its own manual of diagnoses) have relabeled those previously identified with "subjective cognitive complaints" (SCC) as suffering from "subjective cognitive impairment" (SCI). Sutherland *et al.*, in a 2022 article titled, "What Happens to the Worried Well?" found subsequent MCI and dementia in 9 of 166 such "SCI" patients who were followed for up to eight and half years.[95]

Hearing loss (even with the use of hearing aids) is associated with later SCD in men.[97]

Causes of dementia other than AD: Other less common dementia subtypes have a more gradual onset. (See chapter 4).[72]

"Conversion Rates": The Odds of Progression Beyond SCD

The confusing science of odds, rates, and percentages

In this and subsequent chapters, I will often cite numerical results from research studies. In addition to what specific results from individual studies suggest about our futures, what we can take away varies considerably. Much depends on the characteristics of the study's subjects, and how much they resemble you or me.

Reported rates and percentages vary with subject-variables like age, gender, setting (research, community, memory clinic), duration of follow-up, selection criteria, other medical issues, genetics (including country of origin), and context (the body of knowledge at the time the study was conceived).

It is the odds of progression that concerns everyone who has (or thinks they have) SCD. However, for many of us, a discussion of "odds" leads more frequently to thoughts of sports and racetracks rather than cognitive decline. (And we all know how reliable the odds are in sports and gambling.) Even though having SCD is a known *risk* for future dementia,[22] it is not always predictive, and reversal of decline is common.[53,83]

In general, regardless of individual study differences, the odds of developing MCI are consistently greater for those with SCD than for those with no subjective cognitive concerns.[54,83,98-101] Even with that higher risk of progression to MCI and dementia, conversion rates from SCD have been reported as only around 7% per year.[35,100,102] Fifty-three percent of women with subjective complaints developed dementia or MCI versus 38% of controls without complaints.[103]

As with any such study, the total increases with age and the length of time the subjects are followed.[32,58,100] *Importantly, the majority of individuals with subjective cognitive complaints never progress to significant cognitive decline.*[32,83]

The Existence of Cognitive Complaints Does Not Predict Progression to AD

For Alzheimer's disease, specifically, having cognitive concerns is not predictive. When those with memory complaints were tested for the presence of Beta-amyloid, equivalent numbers were positive (55%) or negative (53%).[104] In a large four-year study, equal numbers of individuals (6–7%) with or without SCD at the beginning progressed to dementia.[72] "The course of those with subjective cognitive complaints over time is quite unstable and unpredictable, and these participants can revert to normal cognition."[83] For the development of dementia in those with SCD "the relative risk remains low and SCD cannot be a proxy to preclinical AD."[58]

Predictive (Risk) Factors for Progression from SCD to MCI and/or AD

Clinical factors: Self-perceived cognitive functioning, age, general cognition, and perceived control over future health predicted MCI in 18% of 1,115 SCD subjects.[105] Neuropsychiatric symptoms, including disturbances of mood, perception, and conduct, also have predicted progression to MCI.[98,106,107] "Worried Complainers" (defined as persons whose complaints both impact their activities of daily living, and are noticed by an informant) have the highest risk of progression,[83] up to 2.4 times higher than in the control group.[54,61,108]

The presence of biomarkers increased the likelihood of cognitively unimpaired individuals with SCD progressing to MCI or dementia in a limited number of studies.[32,89,109,110]

Individual characteristics associated with progression include a family history of Alzheimer's disease, mild behavioral impairments, slow gait, depression, rapid weight loss, multiple subtle neurologic abnormalities, vascular disease, and education.[73]

Education: In contrast with the *protection* against AD, which can be acquired through "high educational and occupational attainment," i.e., "cognitive reserve" (chapter 4), the risk of AD associated with SCD is *greater* in highly educated persons, particularly those who perform well on brief (office) cognitive tests like the MMSE.[88,99]

Time-course of progression: As the first stage of decline, SCD can be identified in individuals in their forties. (See Social Demographics, page 40.) When it does devolve into AD, SCD is estimated to predate dementia by ten to fifteen years.[32,45,112]

Evaluation: The first steps for those seeking medical evaluation for SCD should be a medical exam and, potentially, an expanded neuropsychological evaluation.[32] An essential feature of an SCD diagnosis is negative neuropsychological testing.

The goals of testing in SCD are to establish a baseline for the future and to uncover alternative diagnoses for which treatment may be available.

Management: After a clinical evaluation, it's time to bring in others for shared decision-making. When no specific underlying medical or psychiatric condition has been identified, patients with SCD are told to focus on "reassurance, strategies to improve brain health, and annual follow-ups to track any progression."[32]

Common Therapeutic Recommendations

Reassurance that SCD patients do not have AD or MCI is universally mentioned as an "important treatment component."[73] "Reassurance" includes "explaining that (1) SCD is associated with a mildly increased risk of future cognitive decline, particularly in those with so-called SCD-plus features; (2) that SCD can improve spontaneously, and (3) that most individuals with SCD will not experience objective cognitive decline in the near future."[32]

Lifestyle counseling and/or behavioral interventions are often advised to support brain health and emotional well-being, enhance cognition, and decrease conversion to SCD.[72,83] "Treating comorbid conditions: anxiety and depression and reversible causes of cognitive complaints is key to successful outcomes."[73] "Advice should include control of hypertension and diabetes, treatment of mood disorders, physical exercise, weight control, a Mediterranean-style diet, smoking cessation, cognitive and social engagement activities, high-quality sleep, stress reduction, and the use of hearing aids, if needed.[32]"

Some might consider more lifestyle advice "a day late and a dollar short." Basically, this is everything we were repeatedly told to do in the decades before we began forgetting

---

things. Yet, still missing is any guidance specific to memory or cognition. This *is* how we can work on living longer (with or without dementia). Of course, there is nothing wrong with such counsel. All these are accepted public health strategies integral to increasing general health and longevity. But look around—are they working?

Education: An analysis of fifty-six randomized controlled trials of interventions for subjective cognitive decline found that "education programs were most effective for improving memory and cognition." Education was defined as, "a program including several healthy lifestyle strategies such as learning memory strategies, physical conditioning, relaxation techniques and/or diet tips" and offered either in small groups or in books and leaflets.[114]

Annual Follow-up: "Patients with SCI and other risk factors for AD may benefit from annual follow-ups to determine if cognitive problems have progressed to MCI or AD."[73]

What about vitamins, minerals, or supplements? A basic rule is to take nothing that could be harmful in any way or would substitute for proven lifestyle or cognitive interventions. (See chapter 5 for a complete discussion).

SCD treatment is still a work in progress. In their comprehensive review of interventions for subjective cognitive decline, Bhome et al. noted, "There is a lack of high-quality research in this field. Group psychological interventions improve psychological well-being . . . There is no evidence to suggest that cognitive interventions improve global cognitive performance and the clinical utility of small improvements in specific cognitive domains is questionable. There is a lack of research considering lifestyle interventions and poor-quality evidence for pharmacological interventions."[113]

Caution: Those of us with (so far) only self-identified concerns for cognitive decline may be receiving less ongoing medical information. One of my goals is to make us less vulnerable to those offering supplements and other unproven therapies, especially to the extent that they provide one more way of avoiding those annoying "healthy lifestyle choices." Please read the "TO BE AVOIDED" section of chapter 5: Current Treatments for Alzheimer's Disease before trusting your future to jellyfish extract or other medically unsupported remedies. Take the forty-five dollars a month and buy fruit, a gym membership, yoga lessons, or copies of this book for your friends and family.

SCD—Public Health Considerations

Regardless of the presence of measurable cognitive changes, increasing numbers of individuals with subjective decline in cognitive function will seek medical advice.[29,32] The US Centers for Disease Control and Prevention (CDC) considers SCD a public health issue, with the sheer number of those affected an added burden to the healthcare system. Much of the impetus to define, diagnose, and study SCD is because of its implications for millions living with and managing chronic disease, as well as performing everyday activities.

Demographics of SCD: Twenty-nine percent of those diagnosed with SCD live alone. More than two-thirds have two or more chronic diseases, with more than 25% reporting coronary heart disease or stroke. SCD can create the need for assistance in self-management, like help with medications or scheduling medical appointments. Few adults (40% of those sixty-five or older, half of women vs. 39% of men) discuss their memory loss or confusion with health care professionals. The frequency of such discussions also varies with race and ethnicity (46% of Caucasians, 45% of African Americans, 40% of Hispanics, and 34% of Asians and Pacific Islanders.)

A Very Personal Summary of SCD

I am a (self-described) well-read physician, researcher, educator, and author, with enough personal familiarity with dementia to guarantee my ongoing attention to the medical literature. Discovering my own SCD while researching word-finding difficulties and memory lapses was transformative. Most of us are late in life when we acquire new diagnoses. My discovery was a new challenge: first to learn for myself, and then to educate my professional peers and fellow boomers.

SCD is brand new, not yet commonly considered by your primary care physician, and certainly not discussed around the dinner table when we complain about our increasing memory lapses. The extensive use of the current medical model may prevent your doctors from even considering SCD. Instead, you can expect: "Good News! Your office Mini-Mental Status Exam is normal! You're just getting old. See you in a year."

Me: "Hmmm . . . I'd better write that down."

We know from the "odds of progression" above that SCD increases the risk of future cognitive decline. The fact that subjective concerns have been associated with biomarkers means that our personal and private doubts *can* be the first symptomatic stage in the transition to AD.[32,40] Still unrecognized by the International Classification of Diseases and other regulators, SCD was thoroughly examined by an international panel of fourteen experts writing in *Lancet* in 2020.[115] Because it appeared so recently, SCD has not received the extent of research or the level of attention given the other stages of AD. SCD is introduced here because it makes sense to those of us with concerns and because statistically, a percentage of any disease's identified "early" group will progress.

Personally, with aging, I become more apprehensive about speaking. Always respected for my intellect, I now search for words and names with increasing frustration. The good news is that, at least "subjectively," my ability to write clearly, with my full intellectual capacity, is preserved. Maybe it's taking a few more drafts. Word-finding in writing actually can produce better text than my old baseline, as I use the "synonyms" option in my word processor more frequently, and diligently look up names for "that thing that does . . ." on the Worldwide Watchamacallit.

Chapter 3
MILD COGNITIVE IMPAIRMENT (MCI)

Pinning down the best data and guidance for dealing with Subjective Cognitive Decline (chapter 2), is still a work in progress. Advancements are hampered by the SCD syndrome's very nature (only recent awareness, the absence of objective findings, and limited recognition by and attention from the scientific community). This chapter describes the first conclusive findings that can separate those firmly on the threshold of Alzheimer's disease (with a diagnosis of mild cognitive impairment) from the much larger but equally worried population with subjective concerns. What are the tests, and what do they show? What else could it be? What is the likelihood of progressing to dementia, and what can my doctor and I do to improve those odds?

Definition

Mild cognitive impairment (MCI) was the first objectively diagnosed phase of altered cognition preceding Alzheimer's disease. MCI is defined as a slight but measurable decline in office-administered tests of memory and cognition. There is no loss of functional ability.[54,116] MCI is *not* dementia because it does not interfere with everyday activities,[117] but it can progress to dementia, mostly in the form of Alzheimer's disease,[52] the presence of which is defined by biological (biomarker) evidence (chapter 4).

An MCI diagnosis doesn't assure that someone will develop AD, but the odds of progression do increase over time. Investigating a large "early" group for an MCI diagnosis can provide many opportunities for research and intervention before any further deterioration occurs. The MCI label is an "old-school" term. It was created before "waiting for the autopsy" was replaced by sensitive, easily administered tests for biological evidence of Alzheimer's disease. Now, when those diagnosed with MCI biomarkers are found to have brain changes reflecting Alzheimer's disease, they are said to have "MCI due to Alzheimer's disease."

This is yet another page in the expanding portfolio of AD stages. About half of individuals ages sixty-five and older with MCI—roughly 5 million Americans—have MCI due to Alzheimer's disease. Because MCI develops years before dementia and can affect individuals before age sixty-five, many more cases will likely go undiagnosed.[117]

After I recognized the knowledge void surrounding subjective cognitive symptoms, I was motivated to explore MCI by reading that *"more than 80% of Americans know little or are not familiar with mild cognitive impairment (MCI), which can be an early stage in the development of Alzheimer's"* that will likely go undiagnosed. (The Alzheimer's Association, 2021.)[117]

Although a diagnosis of *"mild"* cognitive impairment sounds benign, it is not. If those words have been used to describe you or a loved one, pay extra attention to this chapter. Doctors who deal daily with the full spectrum of dementia say *"mild"* with relief. Patients welcome hearing it, and the word itself makes their exchanges so much easier than at later stages. Alas, there is no stress-free way to say (or hear), "Last stop before Alzheimer's!"

Before biological markers, early stages of AD were identified by their disruption of everyday activities, and by one-on-one neurological testing. The Global Deterioration Scale (GDS) developed in 1982 is still in use today.[118] Like other organizational systems, such scales sort individuals into groups for study. They also clarify communication regarding individual patients.

The Global Deterioration Scale (GDS) description of the clinical characteristics of MCI includes: (1) getting lost while traveling to an unfamiliar location; (2) poor work performance; (3) deficits in word/name finding; (4) retaining little of what is read; (5) decreased facility in remembering names of new people; (6) losing or misplacing an object of value; (7) a concentration deficit on clinical testing.[118]

Other subsequently described clinical signs and symptoms of MCI include:[9,24,118-123]

- Attention deficits, like difficulty following a conversation
- Forgetting intentions upon entering a room
- Increasing dependency on others to fulfill more demanding duties
- Implementing burdensome coping strategies
- Deterioration in visuospatial skills (i.e., disorientation in familiar surroundings, in the absence of underlying motor or sensory disorders)

Rather than coping with memory loss by using common strategies (retracing steps, keeping a diary, maintaining a consistent routine, and having a place for everything), those with MCI tend to cope with memory loss by adopting burdensome coping strategies or increasing their reliance on their partners.[22]

Fortunately, in contrast with dementia, *MCI does not impact the activities of normal living.* "While MCI can make activities of daily living more effortful and challenging, they can be successfully completed independently."[24,32,124,125]

Alas, MCI can lead to complications. "Patients with MCI are at increased risk of delirium (especially during hospitalization), falls, medication errors, and difficulty managing their finances. Older adults with MCI also have increased mortality compared to those with normal cognitive functioning."[9,73]

Word-Finding and Naming Difficulties are Associated With MCI

The inability to find that previously known word now on the "tip of your tongue" (TOT) is one of the most frequently self-acknowledged memory failures. It is that exasperating feeling that accompanies our temporary inability to retrieve information from memory. This is most noticeable with proper nouns (persons, places, or organizations, spelled with an initial capital letter). We "know we know the answer," yet the elusive information is mockingly just outside our mental reach.[126-129] Increasing episodes often heighten concerns about memory decline.

In specific tests of recognizing and recalling the names of famous people from photographs, *TOT has been both associated with and predictive of MCI.*[129-132]

The Two Subtypes of MCI[123]

Amnestic mild cognitive impairment (aMCI) is a clinically significant memory loss that *does not* meet the criteria for dementia. Typically, patients and their families are aware of increasing forgetfulness, but it is not obvious to the casual observer. Cognitive abilities are largely intact.

Non-amnestic mild cognitive impairment (nMCI) is characterized by a subtle decline in functions *not* related to memory (attention, judgment, language, or visuospatial skills). Less common than aMCI, nMCI may precede dementias other than AD.

Neither affects one's independence in activities of daily living.

MCI: "Official" Diagnostic Criteria

The Role of Research

We don't think about medical researchers much, but doctors from the time of Marcus Welby in his home office to "Bones" McCoy on the starship *Enterprise* all rely on the research community to establish precise definitions and diagnostic criteria for most disease states. Only reproducible and objective standards can be used to identify and combine potential research subjects into groups at the same stage of dementia. By following these steps, researchers can begin to adequately describe, quantify, and eventually predict the specific findings unique to that stage. Clinicians can then compare their findings with the descriptions of identified stages to diagnose patients and evaluate treatments.

Diagnostic Criteria

The "official" clinical criterion for a diagnosis of MCI, established by The National Institute on Aging and the Alzheimer's Association (NIA-AA), is *"Cognitive decline from the patient's baseline, as reported by the patient, a knowledgeable informant, or observed by the clinician."* [47,52,124,133]

Additional indicators are:

- Impairment in one or more cognitive domains;
- Cognitive impairment does not interfere with independence in everyday activities;
- The absence of dementia; and

- Individuals can be assigned to one of the two main types, either with or without memory deterioration ("amnestic" (aMCI) or "non-amnestic" (nMCI)).

The American Psychiatric Association (APA), in its *Diagnostic and Statistical Manual of Mental Disorders*, labels patients who have the above criteria for MCI as having "mild neurocognitive disorder." In addition, the APA's "major neurocognitive disorders" list includes all the various dementias listed in chapter 4, with the greatest number of subjects having Alzheimer's disease.[134]

Two patients may walk into different specialists' offices with identical symptoms and the same prognosis. However, the labels they leave with can vary in keeping with the doctor's education and specialty. All of us listen hardest for the encouraging words, and "Mild. . ." sounds pretty good. If your doctor offers a more formal diagnosis, ask for a copy in writing and have someone reliable look it up and discuss it with you.

Neurocognitive Testing and MCI

Alas, Testing for MCI is Unreliable

Many single brief cognitive tests can readily confirm dementia, a presumption that can even be made in social situations or when observing strangers on the street.

However, those routine simple tests for diagnosing dementia are unreliable when the goal is to diagnose MCI, which is defined as "cognitive impairment in the *absence* of dementia."[9,135]

The major issues around testing for MCI include identifying and differentiating MCI from SCD and "normal for age." This is important, since patients with any of these three labels, by definition, can be scored as "normal" on neurocognitive tests. With the standard tests, there is no agreement on the best within-test cutoff points, or even which tests alone can reliably confirm the cognitive decline of MCI.[9] However, one established diagnostic criterion for MCI is identifying "significant changes" from a person's scores on previous administrations of the same tests.

Distinguishing Between MCI and Subjective Cognitive Decline

Similarities between SCD and MCI include a comparable age at onset. Both types of patients will have subjective concerns and complaints, with some inconclusive abnormalities on testing when compared with other groups.

Differentiating MCI from SCD depends on finding reproducible and objective failures on neurocognitive tests that are not found when those with purely subjective concerns are tested. Unfortunately, the usual single, short, easily completed in-office cognitive screening tests (the Mini-Mental Status Examination (MMSE), the Dementia Rating Scale (DRS), and the Montreal Cognitive Assessment (MOCA)) do not clearly differentiate among MCI, SCD, and "normal."[32,52] These in-office tests are best used to identify the final stage, dementia.

Testing for MCI is where the complete half-day set of neuropsychological tests comes in. Those standardized test batteries assess multiple cognitive domains and allow comparisons with age-adjusted, sex-adjusted, and education-adjusted normal scores. Such panels can be repeated over time to identify progression.[52,136-138]

Specific Neurocognitive Tests for MCI

"Batteries" are multiple tests that can be repeated over time and are favored by specialists. Therefore, you may be offered something like Addenbrooke's Cognitive Examinations (ACE). These are short cognitive tests that are widely used to screen for dementia in memory clinics. They distinguish patients with mild aMCI or AD from those with purely subjective concerns.[138-141]

Then, There's DIY ("Do it Yourself") Testing

Test Your Memory for Mild Cognitive Impairment (TYM-MCI): Taking just seven minutes, TYM-MCI successfully separates patients who have passed the MMSE (but were nevertheless suffering from amnestic MCI or mild AD) from normal controls or those with only subjective memory complaints. The TYM-MCI is available to download free for health professionals from tymtest. com. Talk it over with your doctor before going ahead.[139,142-144]

The Self-Administered Gerocognitive Examination (SAGE)[116,145]: This at-home test correlates well with both the classic extensive neuropsychological test battery and the office-administered MMSE. SAGE is more sensitive and specific than the MMSE in differentiating those with cognitive impairment from normal subjects.[145] It may detect MCI conversion to dementia at least six months sooner than MMSE.[146] With the highest validity and reliability of self-administered tools, SAGE can also be administered via electronic devices.[116]

SAGE will not diagnose AD, but it is advocated as a quick tool to identify MCI for anyone concerned about themselves or a loved one.[147] An early MCI diagnosis (which requires that SAGE findings be confirmed by a provider) allows patients and families to be more observant and proactive and can prompt a search for reversible causes of cognitive loss. Getting the jump on social support and financial, legal, and safety needs can improve the long-term quality of life for patients and reduce burdens for their caregivers.[145] SAGE is available at no cost from https ://wexnermedical.osu.edu/brain-spine-neuro/memory

-disorders/sage, requires only paper and pencil, and takes only ten to fifteen minutes. Take it to your doctor for interpretation.

CAUTION: Be sure you want to know and have the resources to cope with the findings. Self-testing is not for everyone and is definitely not advisable for those with no knowledgeable party to consult or without the ability to follow through. Results should be evaluated within an overall medical and psychosocial context, and alternative causes may still need to be ruled out.

Other DIY options include simply counting the number of memory failures noted in diary entries over a week, which was able to distinguish participants with MCI from healthy controls.[148] Tip-of-the-tongue difficulties with proper names may also effectively differentiate MCI patients from normal controls.[130]

The Limitations of Testing

Among the factors that may limit the development of reliable MCI-specific tests is the nature of the control group against whom one's score is compared (their age, demographics, education, IQ, gender, comorbidities, etc.). Every time new research moves the goalpost (defined as a test's cutoff scores for "normal") the proportions of false positive and false negative results change, along with determining how "clinically significant" the various test components and differences are between scores.[138]

The provider's threshold for committing to a diagnosis can be a limiting factor. For example, some clinicians will diagnose MCI based on the presence of only one abnormal result, even though assessing multiple tests can reduce the number of distressing false positive diagnoses.[69]

Since few MCI patients have undergone baseline testing before the onset of their symptoms, clinicians must determine whether a particular score would represent a significant change from a prior one. Such decisions tend to be based on inexact data, and comparisons among a series of subsequent tests will eventually be needed.[9]

"Normal for age" is still what we're all hoping for. Some tests that can distinguish healthy controls from MCI *or* dementia cannot further distinguish between MCI *and* dementia. Unhelpfully, they all get grouped together.

The Role of Alzheimer's Disease (AD) Biomarkers in MCI

Biomarkers can predict decline to AD in patients with MCI, who generally have a greater biomarker load than those with subjective cognitive decline.[69] (For general information on AD biomarkers, see chapter 4)

Risks of biomarker testing for MCI: The likelihood of progression to dementia with a positive biomarker is certainly lower than 100% and is not predictable without ongoing follow-up and testing. Once there's a positive biomarker result, all one can do is worry. Other than providing one more reason to practice good overall health maintenance, *"there is no high quality evidence for, or FDA approval of, pharmacologic treatments for MCI."*[9,149] Positive diagnoses (false-positive or not) are a potential risk to a patient's wellbeing, and adopting unproven treatments can lead to unknown consequences, including heightened states of anxiety, depression, or suicide.

Newer testing modalities: "New" or "early" (and unproven) information is found more readily and in greater quantities than reports of true "scientific breakthroughs." Sources that should be viewed with particular skepticism include the manufacturer's press release; "preliminary," "small," "proof of concept," or "pilot" studies; or an abstract presented at a conference. Wait for FDA approval, peer-reviewed publications, or replication before taking any action.

The news that "new and improved" diagnostic tests are available for sale is frequently released in these ways.

MCI: Prevalence and Risk Factors

The Prevalence of MCI

"A much larger fraction of the population experiences MCI than dementia, and for much longer periods of life."[150] Reported MCI prevalence in older adults varies because of the varying definitions used. Depending on which review you are reading, the estimated MCI prevalence is between 12% and 20% in persons sixty years and older;[151] approximately 7% at ages 60–64 and 25% at ages 80–84.[9,52,149]

Risk factors for—and protective factors against—developing MCI:[52]

- Age: from 10% in those 70–79 years to 25% in those aged 80–89[9]
- Lower levels of education
- Male sex
- Certain personality traits can help one avoid the transition to MCI. Those individuals (particularly females) scoring higher in conscientiousness and extraversion, and lower in neuroticism, lived more years without experiencing cognitive impairment![152]
- Unfortunately, "virtually nothing is known about cultural and racial factors influencing the clinical manifestations of MCI."[9,153]

The Progression of MCI to Dementia

The Evolution from MCI to Alzheimer's Disease

Patients with MCI are almost seven times more likely to develop AD than are older individuals without cognitive impairment.

Reported "conversion rates" from MCI to dementia have varied widely, from 2% to 60% per year.[38] More consistently, 10–15% of individuals with MCI have been thought to progress to AD yearly.[20,146,150,151] When followed for at least three years, rates ranged from 21 to 61%,[146] and after roughly six years 80% are estimated to progress to dementia.

In comparison, *healthy* elderly individuals develop AD at a rate of 1–2% per year.[9] Differences are often attributed to discrepancies in the design of the studies themselves. These include study length, sample size, subject selection criteria, and the tests and definitions applied to the data.

Predictors of progression from MCI to AD:[151,154]

- Older age
- Female gender
- Depression
- Diabetes
- Hypertension
- Severity of impairment on cognitive testing
- Carriers of the apolipoprotein E4 (APOE4) gene
- Brain atrophy
- Abnormal spinal fluid biomarkers. These were associated with subsequent cognitive decline and Alzheimer's-type dementia in 58–79% of MCI patients.[155] When subjects with SCD or MCI and abnormal cerebrospinal fluid (CSF) biomarkers were followed for five years, only 15% remained dementia-free. All of those who reverted to normal cognition had a normal CSF at baseline.[156]

Progression of MCI to AD is Far from Inevitable

Following a diagnosis of MCI, all outcomes still remain possible, including improvement, transition to other forms of dementia, stable deficits that do not progress, and even a recovery to normal cognitive function.[38] In a study of Veterans Administration (VA) patients with "cognitive impairment, not dementia" (equivalent to MCI) over an average of two and a half years, 12% progressed to dementia, 67% continued unchanged, and 21% improved to normal cognition.[157]

The "reversion rate" (from MCI to normal cognition) has been as high as 25 to 30% and is associated with the *absence of spinal fluid biomarkers.*[155,158]

Yes, improvement, and even "reversion," can happen. Reversion has not yet been tied to any specific therapy, is undoubtedly multifactorial, and is unique to each individual and their circumstances. The most likely explanation is the association of improved cognition with the absence of spinal fluid biomarkers (i.e., NOT Alzheimer's).

Not every patient diagnosed with MCI using current cognitive-testing criteria will have the diagnostic anatomic findings of early Alzheimer's disease. (***No amyloid = No AD***) Never become resigned to a future of decline for yourself or a loved one.

Vigorously pursue the numerous other causes of cognitive impairment. (See Differential Diagnosis, immediately below). Follow advances in treatment and caregiving closely and through reliable sources. (See Appendix II.) There is always hope. (See chapter 6.)

The Differential Diagnosis of MCI

The term *differential diagnosis* is used throughout this book. It simply means "other causes"—a list of specific medical conditions that share similar symptoms. The provider's goal is to arrive at the correct diagnosis by eliminating ("ruling out") the other disorders on the differential diagnosis list by using clinical features from the patient's history and exam, as well as the results of necessary testing.

Here's a simple illustration of the concept of "differential diagnosis": Consider a symptom, like cough, that could suggest either a simple upper respiratory infection ("common cold") or a more serious lung infection (pneumonia). Two tests to differentiate between the causes of a cough would be taking a temperature and obtaining a chest X-ray. Both should be normal with a cold and are more likely to be abnormal with pneumonia.

Similarly, "mild" forms of cognitive impairment that may produce "a single abnormal test of cognitive function" are not unique to AD or its precursors. They can be caused by any disorder that creates brain dysfunction, many of which may be treatable, modifiable, or reversible.[146] Common alternative causes of cognitive impairment (the differential diagnosis) include:[9]

Brain disease, injury, or infection: Alzheimer's disease; cerebrovascular disease (stroke); Parkinson's disease; frontotemporal degeneration; adverse central nervous system effects of drugs and toxins; infection; traumatic brain injury; HIV.

Metabolic and endocrine disease: Thyroid disease; vitamin B12 deficiency.

Psychological/Psychiatric disorders: Depression; sleep disorders; chronic psychological stress.

MCI Treatment

No high-quality evidence currently exists to support any drug for the treatment of MCI. Many trials are underway—all with mixed results. For example, some blood-pressure medications have benefited older adults with MCI.[159]

Alzheimer's drugs (see chapter 5): Donepezil has delayed the progression to AD in MCI patients with depression without affecting their depressive symptoms.[9] Cholinesterase inhibitors or memantine, although moderately effective for cognitive symptoms of dementia, do not alter the progression of the disease.[125]

Non-pharmacologic general health improvement measures (see chapter 5) can always help.

PART III: THE DEMENTIAS

Chapter 4
ALZHEIMER'S DISEASE
AND OTHER DEMENTIAS

We began our examination of age-associated cognitive changes with common lapses of information storage and retrieval (memory). Some of us will perceive a loss of cognitive abilities (SCD), and fewer will have their suspicions confirmed by testing (MCI). Few will fail to notice the interference with daily activities that is dementia. Whenever that word is used, we all equate it with Alzheimer's disease (AD), the number one cause. AD is the only dementia type that we regularly hear about (at least until a celebrity publicly acquires one of the others). All dementias are reviewed here, and all are defined by the loss of both memory and cognitive abilities resulting in failure to manage one's basic physical needs. By name, Alzheimer's disease is always "The elephant in the room," with the "room" ranging from the dinner table to the doctor's office to the common areas at the senior center.

Defining Dementia

Dementia is the term used to describe a persistent and disabling decline in cognitive processes (both memory and cognition), leading to the impaired ability to perform essential activities of daily living (ADLs), and culminating in the loss of independence.[24,32,49,73,124] ADLs include bathing or showering, dressing, getting in and out of bed or a chair, walking, using the toilet, and eating.

The American Psychiatric Association (APA), in its latest (2022) *Diagnostic and Statistical Manual of Mental Disorders*[134] categorizes dementia within a group of "Major Neuro-Cognitive Disorders" (MNCDs) These vary in their degree of functional loss. Alzheimer's disease (AD) represents 60–80% of that group.[65]

> Dementia = (Memory Loss)+(Cognitive Loss)+(Interference with Daily Activities)

Alzheimer's Disease: The Basics

By the Numbers

By 2030, an estimated 8.5 million Americans will have Alzheimer's disease, the cause of 75% of dementia in the elderly.[117,124,160,161] By 2050, the US may have more than 13.5 million cases.[65] In 2019, AD was the sixth-leading cause of death for adults in the US (before being surpassed by COVID)[162].

Globally, dementia is the main cause of disability among older adults and is expected to continue to increase as advances allow an increasing fraction of the population to survive to old age. By one estimate, the number of people worldwide living with dementia (36.5 million in 2010) is expected to double every twenty years, with most of those living in low and middle-income countries.[65,163]

Economic burden: The total US health-care costs for Alzheimer's disease and related disorders in 2019 were estimated to be $290 billion. It has been projected to increase to $1.2 trillion in 2050.[164,165]

Alzheimer's Disease: The Essentials

Like other medical conditions, AD is both identified and potentially treated by understanding the biological alterations unique to that diagnosis. At the turn of the nineteenth century, the clinical psychiatrist and neuroanatomist, Alois Alzheimer, had been following a woman in her fifties. For the five years before her death, she was experiencing paranoia, progressive sleep and memory disturbances, and aggression. At her autopsy, using new methods of staining brain cells for examination, Alzheimer identified the hallmark lesions of AD in specific brain regions:

(1) "neuritic plaques" of abnormal nerve cells composed of beta-amyloid protein,
(2) unusual fiber clusters of tau proteins in the cerebral cortex ("neurofibrillary tangles"), and
(3) an associated loss of normal brain cells ("neurodegeneration").

Alzheimer described the anatomical changes in his patient's brain to a 1906 conference as "A Peculiar Severe Disease Process of the Cerebral Cortex," later labeled "Alzheimer's disease."[166] When absorbed in body fluids, these abnormal proteins (beta-amyloid and tau) cause AD, likely by directly injuring brain cells. It is these abnormal proteins that define AD as unique among the various other neurodegenerative disorders that can lead to dementia.[65,125]

The Genetic Basis of AD (see also "Unmodifiable Risk Factors," below)

Approximately 70% of the risk of developing AD can be attributed to genetics.[65,167-169]

The fundamental genetics of inheritance: Two categories of genes influence whether a person will develop an inheritable disorder:[170]

"Causative genes" produce a disease. Three of these (APP, PSEN1, and PSEN2) directly induce the rare early-onset form of AD. Different genes cause other serious neurologic conditions, like Huntington's disease.

"Risk genes" are the second category. They don't initiate the disease, but they do increase the likelihood of developing it under specific conditions. Alzheimer's disease is associated with variations in multiple risk genes, as are other common neurologic conditions such as multiple sclerosis (MS) and Parkinson's disease.

Family history: Before specific genes could be identified, family histories provided the earliest evidence for inherited factors in AD.[171] In families, the age of disease onset defines two distinct mechanisms of inheritance.

(1)　Early-onset Alzheimer's disease (EOAD) is found in only 1–5% of all Alzheimer's patients but is responsible for half of the small number of AD cases that occur before age sixty. EOAD "runs in families" resulting from autosomal dominant inheritance of one of the three causative genes. Alzheimer's is found in approximately half the children in each EOAD generation, and an affected child typically has an affected parent.

(2)　Late-onset Alzheimer's disease (LOAD): Ninety-nine percent of AD cases are late-onset, occurring in individuals over age sixty-five. More commonly referred to as "sporadic" AD, LOAD is highly "heritable" (meaning readily passed on from parents to children, but without a particular genetic mechanism or obvious familial pattern, i.e., not dominant or recessive). LOAD heritability accounts for the two-to-threefold increased risk of developing AD in first-degree relatives (siblings or children) of AD patients.

Except for the difference in inheritance (familial vs. sporadic), once manifested, both forms of AD behave the same clinically.

Typical AD symptoms and course: Waning memory with age was noted as long ago as 700 B.C.[172] Alzheimer's discovery of amyloid plaques and tangles of tau protein in his patient's brain *anatomically* defined Alzheimer's disease. However, it remains the observable day-to-day changes in cognition, memory, and behavior that *affirm* the clinical syndrome of Alzheimer's dementia.

Typically, as we experience AD in our families, friends, and associates, the clinical profile is one of progressive memory loss, particularly early failures of short-term memory. Other common signs involve language, loss of visuospatial abilities (like drawing, buttoning a shirt, making a bed), diminished executive functions (like impulse and emotional control, planning, prioritization, and problem-solving), and a shrinking working memory (that small amount of information which can be held temporarily in mind and is needed to execute cognitive tasks).

Those affected may or may not be aware of their cognitive deficits. Failing memory and cognitive functions lead to significant disruptions in daily life, like forgetting conversations and plans, difficulty with finances, disorientation to time and place, and frequently misplacing items.

Along with these cognitive features, several neuropsychiatric symptoms appear. Irritability, apathy, and depression are common in the early stages, with delusions and hallucinations occurring more frequently later. Sleep disruption, which can be distinctly different from or just more severe than typical age-related changes, is common, with the degree of poor sleep correlating with brain amyloid burden.[173]

Dementia can be associated with adverse financial events years before its appearance. These become more prevalent after diagnosis and were most common in census tracts with lower levels of education. Examples include missed payments on credit accounts and falling credit scores.[174] Other key features of AD are its insidious onset, gradual progression, and a characteristic pattern of deficits.[65,175]

Clinically Defined Stages of AD: As in almost any slowly progressive disease (cancer comes to mind), there is an undetectable ("preclinical") silent phase. The illness is just taking hold and no overt changes are noticeable. At the far end of the progression is the very characteristic late phase of Alzheimer's disease, when dysfunction is prominent and the diagnosis is most easily made. In the intermediate stages (SCD and MCI) when milder changes are present, the diagnosis can be considered, some diagnostic measures become abnormal, and progression occurs.[17]

The Global Deterioration Scale: In 1982, after four years of systematic observations of patients, Reisberg and his associates published the Global Deterioration Scale (GDS). It remains in wide use today.[176,177] The GDS describes seven distinct observable phases in the clinical evolution of the AD syndrome. At the time, the presence of those observable stages would support a diagnosis of "probable Alzheimer's disease."

Categorizing the progression of a disease by numbering stages of increasing severity is regularly seen in medicine, particularly in cases of serious illnesses. Doing so provides a common descriptive language and shorthand.

Such clinical descriptions of the stages of a progressive disease allow us to visualize, summarize, and communicate where an individual or group of patients appear on the spectrum of a complex disorder. Researchers can identify and cluster similar groups of patients for study. Agreed-upon labels for stages get everyone on the same page. Stages clarify communications among providers and with patients and families. Long-term observations of larger identified subgroups can facilitate predictions for an individual's course and potential response to therapies.[121,177,178] Knowing where a loved one is on a foreseeable trajectory empowers families to plan for what is likely coming—however intimidating.

The Global Deterioration Scale (GDS) includes:

GDS 1 — no subjective complaints of memory deficit and no memory deficit on clinical interview.

GDS 2 — subjective complaints of memory deficits with no objective deficits in employment or social situations. (GDS 2 is equivalent to subjective cognitive decline, chapter 2.)

(Since 2011, stages 1 and 2 have been classified as "preclinical" (unverifiable) Alzheimer's disease.)[179]

GDS 3 — the earliest clear-cut deficit with objective evidence on detailed interview and decreased performance in demanding employment and social settings (mild cognitive impairment, chapter 3).

GDS 4 — a clear-cut deficit after a careful clinical interview manifests in such areas as decreased knowledge of current and recent events and concentration deficits on serial subtractions, with decreased ability in the performance of complex tasks such as managing finances or preparing dinner for guests.

GDS 5 — a deficit sufficient to interfere with independent community survival, and the inability to recall a major relevant aspect of current and past life during the clinical interview (e.g., address or telephone number of many years or names of certain close family members, or the names of schools attended for years and from which they may have graduated).

GDS 6 — a deficit sufficient to require assistance with basic activities of daily life such as dressing and bathing with a general lack of awareness regarding recent events and life experiences and sketchy knowledge of personal history.

GDS 7 — a deficit sufficient to require assistance with toileting and feeding, with both urinary and fecal incontinence, and with severely circumscribed or entirely absent verbal abilities and, ultimately, loss of ambulatory skills.[176]

Moving from Clinical Description to Objective Testing and a Research Agenda

Newer studies of Alzheimer's disease's progression have added objectivity and consistency by including scores from neurocognitive testing along with observation and self-report. As a result, the depiction of AD has progressed from the original narrative by Alzheimer in 1906,[166] past Reisberg's seven stages,[177] to include the sixty-five thousand citations with "Alzheimer's disease" in the title listed in the National Library of Medicine database (PubMed) in February 2023.

Between 2015 and 2019 multiple prestigious sources (from major textbooks to the World Health Organization,[180,181] the National Academies of Sciences, and others), all similarly described the progression from "normal" levels of age-related cognitive decline to dementia.[5,17,47,49,65,149,182,183]

The consensus was that the earliest identification of AD depended on a diagnosis of MCI defined by scores on standard neurocognitive tests below those of age-matched "normal controls"[9] or the presence of overt dementia. Those with no symptoms or subjective symptoms only, and normal neurocognitive testing (e.g., subjective cognitive decline, chapter 2) were not, at that time, classified as at risk for AD, or reliably differentiated from the "worried well" with their "senior moments."

Biomarkers: The Biological Basis of an AD Diagnosis

The Influence of Biomarkers on the Evolving Study of Alzheimer's Disease

For the longest time, AD could only be definitively diagnosed after death by a history of dementia combined with characteristic brain lesions (amyloid plaques) found at autopsy.[65] A dilemma arose when it became clear that dementia is only the highly visible late stage of a disorder that takes years to develop silently in the brain. To study AD and its progression, one must first find, then study and research subjects at the earliest phase of the disease, ideally when memory and cognition are still "normal for age" (the "preclinical" stage).

The existence of asymptomatic Alzheimer's disease was first confirmed when cognitively normal individuals were found to have AD pathology on postmortem examination of their brains. In fact, approximately 60%–98% of adults over sixty with *no* signs of cognitive impairment during life will have changes of AD in their brains at the time of their death.[58,184-187]

Research expanded dramatically when *in vivo* (Latin for "within the living") tests using brain-imaging or body-fluid analysis replaced autopsies to diagnose AD. Using these physical or chemical "biomarkers," investigators found the amyloid and tau proteins of underlying AD in approximately 30% of *cognitively normal* older adults! Such positive biomarkers in the absence of cognitive changes result in the diagnosis of preclinical Alzheimer's disease.[30,49,179,187-189]

Biomarkers allow estimates of the size of the population in pre-dementia stages of Alzheimer's disease. The first worldwide estimates using biomarker techniques was 69 million individuals with mild cognitive impairment (MCI) due to AD in 2022 and more than 300 million individuals with preclinical AD as of 2019.[190]

Mild cognitive impairment (MCI, chapter 3), the first identifiable precursor of Alzheimer's disease, is still diagnosed by cognitive test scores below the expected range for that individual.[124] Along with the final stages of dementia, which could always be identified clinically, these two earlier stages (preclinical and MCI) reflect the common understanding of AD progression when the most recent academic knowledge summaries were published (2015-19).[133] Subjective cognitive decline (SCD, chapter 2) came later. A suggested framework for the study of SCD was published in 2014,[92] but its characteristics were not fully described until 2020.[32]

Biomarkers Become Equated with the Diagnosis of AD

In establishing diagnostic criteria for AD, biological markers are distinguished from those clinical tools (interviews, tests, questionnaires, memory tasks) that identify and quantify the cognitive and behavioral markers of dementia. Techniques for detecting AD biomarkers vary in invasiveness, availability, complexity, specificity, cost, and acceptance by the medical community. The test characteristic that matters to doctors and patients is simple. *Does the test identify the presence of the amyloid or tau proteins that are the direct cause of Alzheimer's dementia?* By replacing autopsy as the most reliable evidence of the brain changes causing AD, brain scans and body-fluid analysis both narrowed the official benchmarks for diagnosing AD and widened the availability of early and definitive answers.

The ability to definitively diagnose AD before death, along with the less costly and less invasive tests for those markers, converted the previously invisible state of preclinical Alzheimer's disease from an assumption into a verifiable diagnosis. The International Working Group (IWG) advising both major organizations funding Alzheimer's research re-defined preclinical Alzheimer's disease as *"the stage at which a biomarker of AD pathology is present, but symptoms have not yet developed."*[32] The diagnosis of AD was no longer limited to those with observable failings of memory and cognition but is now defined in living persons solely by the *presence of biological changes.* These advances make the much larger number of persons in the earliest (preclinical) stage available for study and can guide or eliminate further study for those who test negative. The majority of the estimated 47 million people who are in this preclinical phase of AD are under the age of seventy.[191]

The assumption is that the sooner AD can be diagnosed, the earlier approved treatments can be applied to potentially delay or even prevent the clinical AD syndrome.[32,192] We have now come full circle: the diagnosis returns to the anatomic focus of the disease discovered by Alzheimer in his patient's brain over a century ago.

Although the presence of biomarkers defines preclinical Alzheimer's disease, it does not predict dementia. As with any complex disorder, AD, even when clearly identifiable biologically, can still vary widely in its manifestations, from cognitively normal to dementia. Rising biomarker levels have been documented in middle-aged persons cognitively normal at baseline and followed for up to a decade. The greater the rate of change, the more likely the development of MCI.[193] The proportion of cognitively normal older adults with brain-scan changes of AD increases with age, from 10% at age fifty to 44% by age ninety.[187] Preclinical AD has been found (whether measured at autopsy or *in vivo*) in the roughly 30% of older adults who "have brains littered with enough amyloid or tau, or both to qualify for an Alzheimer's diagnosis but are without so much as a hint of dementia."[30,194,195]

Biomarkers and the clinical staging of AD: The Global Deterioration Scale of Reisberg and associates described earlier remains an accurate picture of the typical clinical course of AD (ranging from the absence of any subjective or objective abnormalities (GDS 1) to the loss of speech and ambulation (GDS 7). The current labeling of decline towards dementia also tracks the brain changes causing the disease,[124] with a smaller proportion of the elderly ending up in each successive stage.[196]

Which AD-Specific Biomarkers Are Available?[197,198]

Brain imaging: The ability to detect AD by noninvasive brain imaging was the first breakthrough in *in vivo* definitive diagnosis. Subsequent developments allowing measurements of brain-cell metabolic activity and the degree and location of atrophy (neurodegeneration) became powerful aids to diagnosis, staging, and prognosis. This is particularly important because such changes begin to appear up to twenty to thirty years before clinical dementia.[50,54,58,65,72,187,194,199-202] Brain imaging biomarkers include:[198]

(1) Computed tomography (CT). While this is the least sensitive scan, it takes only a few minutes and can be particularly useful in identifying non-Alzheimer's causes of dementia like tumors, stroke, and head injury. CT scans *will* show the shrinkage of brain regions that may occur with dementia. However, they are poor at tracking changes over time. More specialized procedures (such as

single-photon emission computed tomography, or
SPECT-CT) can reveal blood flow abnormalities
associated with various dementia syndromes.[203]

(2) MRI uses magnetic fields and radio waves to
produce detailed images of the volume, size and
shape of the brain and its various regions. Repeat
scans will reveal changes over time.[198]

(3) PET (Positron Emission Tomography) adds small
amounts of injected radioactive tracers to CT
scanning to detect changes in biochemical activity
in specific brain regions. Using different tracers,
PET scans identify deposits of amyloid-beta or tau
proteins. *A negative amyloid-PET scan rules out most
forms of AD*. Failing brain areas can be detected
by their decreased uptake of glucose (FDG-
PET). Amyloid and tau PET scans are commonly
employed to definitively identify individuals with
AD for research. They can then be repeated to
assess the impact of experimental drugs.

Brain imaging is also used to validate the accuracy of body-
fluid biomarkers used in AD clinical trials.[204] While the predictive powers of more sophisticated scans continue to evolve,[201,202]
imaging fails in the diagnosis of some non-Alzheimer dementias like chronic traumatic encephalopathy (CTE) which still
requires autopsy specimens and a microscope.

Cerebrospinal fluid (CSF), which bathes the brain and spinal cord, is examined to identify and quantify abnormal proteins released from amyloid and tau.[50,54,65,201,205,206] Changes in
CSF markers have also been shown to occur decades before the
onset of clinical AD.[58]

When offered CSF biomarker testing, patients and families
need to understand that CSF is obtained via lumbar puncture
(LP), commonly referred to as a "spinal tap," and a thorough

risk/benefit assessment should take place. There is no question that LP can be a critical and even life-saving technique to identify causes of mental status changes at any age. However, be aware that the risks and discomforts of LP escalate significantly with the physical limitations imposed by aging, as well as the problems of obtaining the necessary cooperation and consent in those with agitation, dementia, or other mental status changes.

The figure below illustrates lumbar puncture in a young person. Imagine how difficult this would be to perform safely on your loved one, or anyone old, frail, agitated, or confused. Adding sedation greatly multiplies the risks of the procedure in the elderly: vomiting, aspiration, and introducing one more powerful drug that could cause a negative reaction.

Lumbar Puncture

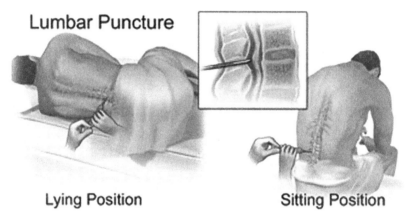

Lying Position   **Sitting Position**

Lumbar puncture is the procedure of placing a
hollow needle into the lower back between the bones
of the spine to remove some cerebrospinal fluid (CSF),
usually for diagnostic purposes.

As an alternative to LP, Amyloid PET scans are considered "highly concordant" (80%–90% agreement) with CSF in predicting amyloid positivity.[58] Alas, even scans in the agitated elderly will often require sedation, with associated risks.

Simply testing blood for AD proteins would certainly be familiar, desirable, and easily tolerated. However, many such tests are still early in their development and often are more appropriately intended for "research purposes only."[207-210]

The PrecivityAD™ test,[211] at $1,250 (and not covered by insurance)[212]is the first *publicly* available blood test for AD, measuring both plasma amyloid and the APOE gene.[213] Like all laboratory tests, its accuracy depends on a scientifically valid relationship between the characteristics of the population on which the test was developed and those to whom it is later applied in practice. For example, a patient's race can significantly affect a plasma biomarker's detection of amyloid.[214]

No test is reliable when it is used outside the medical context for which it was developed. As an example, if you gave an approved pregnancy test to enough men, some would return (falsely) positive. While *those* test failures would be easy to identify, false-positive results wrongly interpretable as asymptomatic (preclinical) Alzheimer's disease, are not.

Despite the relative ease, familiarity, and increasing availability of Alzheimer's blood testing, receiving positive results will be life-changing. Therefore, the recommendation for the use and interpretation of results should only come from an expert clinician after a full evaluation. "Standalone use . . . carries a significant risk of misinterpretation and is strongly discouraged."[215]

Newer and better tests will continue to emerge, and combinations of tests may yield higher degrees of accuracy.[189,216] Artificial intelligence, combined with a novel genetic blood test, may one day detect and predict AD.[217]

The ATN scoring system is successful in differentiating between individuals with AD and controls. ATN sorts patients into groups based on which of the eight possible patterns of positive and negative results they demonstrate after testing for beta-amyloid (**A**), pathological tau (**T**), and the degree of brain-cell damage (neurodegeneration, **N**).[49,201,218] Positive results for both amyloid and tau (A+/T+), or amyloid marker-positive and tau-pathology negative (A+/T-) define Alzheimer's disease. Amyloid marker-negative and tau pathology-positive (A-/T+) results will identify the absence of Alzheimer's disease.[32]

Measurement of bodily functions as biomarkers: Olfactory dysfunction (changes in the sense of smell) was found to be a biomarker for degeneration of brain cells detectable by imaging. A single abnormal measurement predicted cognitive decline up to fifteen years later. It also predicted an increased risk of conversion from normal cognition to MCI and AD. The more rapid the olfactory decline, the higher the risk.[219]

Of interest, a persistent loss of the sense of smell after COVID-19 was a better predictor of long-term cognitive and functional impairment ("brain fog") than the severity of the initial disease.[220]

Biomarker Limitations

As was true over a hundred years ago, there is strong evidence of the abnormal transformation of brain cells in AD. Such changes are now found early in brain images and body fluids instead of at an autopsy. These biomarkers clearly define AD and underlie its manifestations.

"Positive biomarkers = AD"[49]

Biomarkers create diagnostic certainty and the ability to follow the footprints of AD in living patients, including unimpaired individuals in the preclinical stage. As with any test or treatment, the decision to employ biomarkers to assess patients with cognitive concerns or findings offers both risks and benefits (see also chapter 6). Unlike in the research setting, expensive, uncomfortable, or investigational tests should rarely be the first step in the evaluation of patients with memory complaints or cognitive difficulties. Like many entities in medicine, AD is initially suspected from a pattern of clinical findings. Such an informed, but unconfirmed, diagnosis should likely be termed, *"probable or possible Alzheimer's disease."*

Once the "A-word" is used, it can't be revoked. Such labeling should originate from those with a higher level of diagnostic skill than lab results from a website, or cousin Bob saying, "Dad is acting just like Uncle Harvey before he started the fire in the bathroom; we'd better start looking for a nursing home."

Unfortunately, when based solely on failings in cognition, memory, and behavior, diagnoses of "possible or probable AD or Alzheimer's syndrome" lack both sensitivity and specificity. "This is AD, I know it when I see it" hardly inspires trust in the result! A pattern of purely clinical features, like "probable Alzheimer's disease" is a description that can fit several diseases. (See the differential diagnosis of dementia syndromes below.)

The presence of a clinical syndrome does not "rule *in* the pathologic changes of AD—nor does the absence of the syndrome rule it *out.*" In fact, 10% to 30% of individuals clinically diagnosed as having Alzheimer's dementia will not display AD pathology on scans, spinal fluid testing, or autopsy.[49]

Confusion between the behavioral syndrome and the anatomic disease can lead to communication difficulties between doctors and families. In the absence of biomarker evidence, such confusion can result in premature diagnostic closure with the associated failure to consider other less common diagnoses, some with available treatments or with radically different implications for both patient and family.

For example, in their 2022 textbook *Memory Loss, Alzheimer's Disease, and Dementia*, Budson and Solomon[43] noted that in the days before biomarker testing,

> After evaluating a patient, we might make a clinical diagnosis of Alzheimer's disease dementia, knowing that we were likely to be correct when the patient came to autopsy 80% to 90% of the time. We, therefore, would communicate the diagnosis of 'probable Alzheimer's disease' to the patient and family in an honest and confident manner, and then segue into discussions about treatment.
>
> Although the clinical diagnosis would be incorrect 10% to 20% of the time, this *misdiagnosis* [emphasis added] would only come to light at autopsy—which few patients would receive. Relying only on a clinical diagnosis of Alzheimer's syndrome, patients without biomarker confirmation are often treated with drugs only approved for Alzheimer's disease, regardless of their underlying pathology. *Today, although our clinical accuracy is still 80% to 90% . . . we are now faced [because of biomarker availability] with telling 1-2 of every 10 patients that that the diagnosis was wrong, and they don't have Alzheimer's disease.* This may be understandably upsetting, particularly given the discomfort, delays, and expense of biomarker tests.[124]

Whether or not to open the door to biomarker testing is a serious decision that will vary widely among currently unaffected older adults, their doctors, and their families.

The Potential Consequences of Knowing One's Biomarker Status

Those with positive AD biomarkers do worse than their peers without them.[30] In cognitively unimpaired individuals over sixty, the larger the brain biomarker load (amyloid or tau), the greater the severity of their cognitive concerns[32] and the risks of progression.[58] Tests continue to improve and multi-test "panels" and other novel analytical platforms are in development to detect and predict AD before symptoms appear.[138-141,218]

We're getting there, slowly. Early detection is a big part of the solution. Timely diagnosis will hopefully lead to more personalized care and "effective management in the absence of an effective drug."[198] Prevention and treatments before deficits develop are still far in the future.

Predicting "lifetime risk": One goal of biomarker research is to acquire enough data on asymptomatic individuals to make predictions with confidence, both for individuals and for the populations they represent. Ideally, one might someday be able to say: "With this positive test you have a ___% likelihood of progressing to ____within ____ years"; or "a treatment that extends cognitive abilities for ten years will produce the following social and economic benefits. . . " Based on age, gender, biomarker tests for preclinical disease, and historical death rates, it is now possible to model an individual's "lifetime risk of developing AD dementia." For example, the lifetime risk of AD for a ninety-year-old female who is only positive for amyloid is 8.4% (5.4% for a male). For a sixty-five-year-old woman with the same results, the lifetime risk of AD is 29.3% (22% for a male). Those younger than eighty-five years old with mild cognitive impairment, amyloidosis, and neurodegeneration have lifetime risks of AD dementia greater than 50%. The model also provides information about shorter-term risks of progression; for example, a sixty-five-year-old white female with amyloidosis and neurodegeneration has a 41% lifetime risk of developing AD, but only a 10.7% chance within the next ten years.[191]

Using this model, *of the estimated 46.7 million Americans currently living with preclinical AD, 12.6 million (27%) of them will develop clinical AD.* Of course, these are population-based estimates with no current way to identify the specific one in four of those 47 million who will progress.

The good news from this model: ***Most persons (73%) with preclinical AD will not develop Alzheimer's dementia during their lifetimes.***

Based on what is currently known, it is likely true that a majority of those with preclinical AD will not progress. A statistical model like this is basically a "black box" filled with computer code, advanced mathematics, and programmer assumptions, being fed large numbers from various sources. As new data is entered, outputs will change. Conclusions here are particularly influenced by the key denominator—the actual number of cases of preclinical AD. This will vary widely with the population studied and could only truly be known if everyone is tested.

Predicting the onset of symptoms is possible. Serial measurements of single and combined tests have recently recognized very specific threshold levels of biomarker results that can predict a period of rapid escalation in the build-up of AD proteins. Such methods offer the ability to forecast when cognitively normal individuals with brain amyloidosis will develop symptoms of Alzheimer's disease, pinpointing a specific time frame for action. Such a "tipping point in amyloid accumulation" was found on repeated positron emission tomography (PET) amyloid scans[221], as well as with recurrent combined amyloid PET and cerebrospinal fluid (CSF) sampling.[222]

The age of symptom onset was found to strongly correlate with the age at which an individual reaches this tipping point.[221] *These findings suggest a future when patients could potentially be informed not just "if," but "when" they might develop dementia.*[223]

Here is good news for those who choose to know their biomarker status: *negative predictive value is high.* False positive CSF biomarker tests are particularly rare, illustrating that one valuable clinical use of biomarker testing may be for reassurance.[72]

General Biomarker Caveats

"It's complicated." From biomarkers, we learned that it is unusual for a patient to have a single biological failure responsible for cognitive impairment. Most patients have at least two and many have three or more contributing factors.[224] Biomarker positivity alone is not yet a sufficient predictor of clinical AD or its degree. While positive biomarkers mean you have the biological basis for AD, that does not mean that any symptoms you are having are due to that disease, or that you will develop symptoms of AD in the future.[49]

Research on age groups can indeed determine *collective* probabilities of progression over time. However, even in the "age of biomarkers" a single individual's chances of moving from absentminded to out-of-it remain unpredictable, with only a modest correlation between markers and the extent of clinical dementia.[201]

Multiple studies note the presence of biomarkers in neurologically healthy control subjects, with a prevalence of 14–67%.[225] However, the additional presence of a marker of tau pathology is associated with a more rapid progression to clinical

AD, suggesting that the presence of both can better define AD, while amyloid positivity alone may not be sufficient.[58,187]

The use of biomarkers to diagnose AD in the absence of clinical findings has been called into question by the very body that initially suggested that such markers should serve as the "biological definition of Alzheimer's disease" in 2018.[49] In 2021, the NIA-AA International Working Group (IWG) reviewed the use of purely biological means, originally intended for research, to diagnose AD in everyday clinical practice. When they considered the limitations of biomarkers in the diagnosis of Alzheimer's disease, the Working Group concluded that "emerging studies suggest that *the biomarker definition is not ready for application in clinical settings and for diagnosis of individuals without cognitive impairment.*" The IWG now recommends that an "Alzheimer's disease diagnosis be restricted to people who have positive biomarkers together with specific Alzheimer's disease phenotypes [observable clinical characteristics]. However, *biomarker-positive cognitively unimpaired individuals should be considered only "at-risk for progression to Alzheimer's disease."*[226]

Brain imaging caveats: Brain imaging plays a very significant role, particularly when differentiating AD from other causes of dementia. Some findings are not specific to AD, but indicate damage that may derive from various causes, such as stroke. Imaging can supplement body-fluid biomarkers. For example: CSF markers report the concentrations (percentages) of AD-specific proteins in spinal fluid on a specific date, but these fluctuate day to day. On the other hand, imaging measures reflect the totality of accumulated brain-structure damage.[49]

Comorbidities may cloud the interpretation of some biomarkers: The majority of brains from patients with dementia attributed to AD also exhibit varying amounts of cerebrovascular disease or abnormal proteins unrelated to AD. "The degree to which a given patient's cognitive impairments can be attributed to one pathology or another is hard to know."[201]

The Biomarker Bottom Line

With continual refinements, the antemortem determination of AD pathology in people with or without dementia is much improved, now with 89% to 100% accuracy.[201] Markers are useful for: (1) confirming AD at later stages of dementia, (2) the earliest detection of a tendency to develop AD, and (3) narrowing the differential diagnosis of a dementia. Findings suggest a twenty-to-thirty-year interval between the first development of amyloid positivity and the onset of dementia.[187]

The "worried well" may find little reassurance in the science of biomarkers. We older folks, or our families, will be motivated by even "normal for age" cognitive decline to seek more information and the promise of hope. The difference between "normal" aging and other diagnoses is the probability of progression to MCI/AD. Regardless of the caveats above, the sheer number of worried elderly represents a huge market for tests offering to pin down the likelihood of progressive cognitive decline. In fact, it's the same large audience for whom this book is intended.

The Six NIA-AA Stages of AD and their Descriptions

The current formal designations of AD stages are those adopted by the working group from the National Institute on Aging and the Alzheimer's Association (NIA-AA). As discussed earlier, the first description, in 2018, was a *biomarker-based* "research framework" and "biological definition" of Alzheimer's disease.[49] While the most recent analysis, in 2021, focused on "clinical diagnosis," [226] the original six NIA-AA numeric stages reflecting increasing severity of the disease have not been replaced.[32,196]

The Six NIA-AA Stages of Alzheimer's Disease

Stage 1: No symptoms or subjective or objective concern about for cognitive decline.

Stage 2: The transitional stage—individuals with the first subtle signs of AD: Subjective cognitive decline (SCD), or subtle objective cognitive decline, without criteria for impairment. Recent onset mild behavioral symptoms could co-occur or could be the predominant symptom.

Stage 3: MCI (chapter 3). Objective cognitive impairment short of dementia:

(a) Cognitive decline with impairment;
(b) Mild functional impairment possible; or
(c) Independence preserved.

Stages 4, 5, and 6: Alzheimer's disease with mild, moderate, or severe dementia.

Evidence Required for Staging Alzheimer's Disease

Staging can also be based on associations between when symptoms occur and the presence of biomarkers. All patients can be divided into (1) those with and without symptoms, including either or both subjective or objective (neurocognitive testing abnormalities) findings and (2) those who are or are not positive for an AD biomarker. Identifying patients at the asymptomatic stage is the foundation for preventive approaches.

See Table 1:

Table 1: Evidence Required for Staging Alzheimer's Disease

	DIAGNOSTIC STAGES OF AD*				
	"Normal for Age"	Preclinical AD	SCD	MCI	AD***
Subjective Symptoms	–	–	+	+	+
Neurocognitive Testing	–	–	–	+	+
Biomarkers**	–	+	+	+	+
Percent Progressing to AD	10% Men, 20% Women	27%	54%	80%	--------
Reference:	227	228	54	9	--------

* **SCD** = Subjective symptoms only;
MCI = Neurocognitive test failure only;
AD = Alzheimer's Dementia

**Biomarkers may not always be obtained, but presence of a unique marker of AD in brain, blood, or cerebrospinal fluid 100% defines the presence of AD.

***Biomarker-positive (+) and Symptoms–negative (-) equals Alzheimer's disease in waiting!

The Stages and Progression to AD

A dwindling percentage of patients in the earlier stages progress to Alzheimer's disease. Not surprisingly, the probability of progression increases with age. The transition from normal cognition to MCI due to AD ranged from 4% to 10% annually. If you are age sixty-five, the annual rate of change to a more severe stage varies with your current cognitive status. Eight percent of sixty-five-year-olds with normal cognition are likely to worsen in a year. The odds increase for those of us entering Medicare age who already have cognitive decline: 22% for those with MCI due to AD, and 25%, 36%, and 16% for groups with pre-existing mild, moderate, or severe AD respectively. Worsening cognitive impairment and increased age both add to the likelihood of institutionalization and death.[196]

Beyond Stages

The usefulness of thinking of AD in terms of discrete stages has evolved into the concept of a *"continuum."*[49,58] Both cognitive decline and biomarker progression in AD occur *continuously* over a prolonged period that begins before symptoms. The scientific community now views Alzheimer's as a spectrum of disease. The stages range from an asymptomatic (but biomarker-positive) preclinical phase to subjective symptoms of decline (SCD, chapter 2), then mild cognitive impairment (MCI, chapter 3), and finally, dementia (AD, chapter 4)[30]

The preclinical stage progresses imperceptibly. Clinical manifestations eventually appear, but without a well-defined onset. Progressive biological changes correlate with increasingly severe clinical stages of the disorder.

Neurocognitive Testing

Historically, Alzheimer's Disease Was a "Diagnosis of Exclusion"

Prior to biomarkers and excluding autopsy, there was little objective testing available to confirm a diagnosis. AD was identified by going down the list of dementias (see below) and clinically excluding the other possibilities. This process is common in medicine when a diagnosis cannot be confidently established from history, examination, or testing.

In the past, when someone developed slowly progressive memory loss with some cognitive impairment and all major alternative explanations were excluded, the likelihood of AD as the culprit was considered high, and a "clinical diagnosis was made." When compared with postmortem confirmations, the accuracy of such pre-death clinical diagnoses was only considered "modest." Sensitivities ranged from 71% to 87% and the specificity from 44% to 71%.[201]

The "Sensitivity" and "Specificity" of Tests Can Be Confusing

"Sensitivity" refers to a test's ability to identify an individual with a disease as having a positive result. A highly sensitive test means that there are few false negative results, and thus fewer cases of disease are missed.

The specificity of a test is its ability to designate an individual who does not have a disease as negative, limiting false positives.

The Role of Neurocognitive Testing in AD Diagnosis[58]

Before biomarkers were available to confirm the presence of the underlying physiology and anatomy of AD, neurocognitive testing identified the onset of clinical AD by observing "sustained and significant declines over time" in scores from repeated tests of cognition, memory, or combinations of the two.

When large groups of cognitively healthy subjects are followed over time with traditional tests, differences in scores between those who will eventually develop dementia and those who will not, can be observed ten to seventeen years before a final dementia diagnosis. At a group level, cognitive changes initially consist of subtle, small decreases in scores of episodic memory (conscious memory of a previous experience), psychomotor speed (the time to process information and respond physically to it), verbal fluency, and concept formation.

Caution: Declining test scores are not specific to, or predictive of, AD. They can also be seen in other conditions such as depression, substance use disorder, and Parkinson's disease.

Single Tests For Dementia[206]

Traditional, formal neurocognitive evaluations are interpreted by a specialist, cover a dozen or more categories of cognitive behavior, and can take up to a full day. Single tests for dementia are frequently used in primary care settings. While they provide no biological confirmation, their short administration times and satisfactory sensitivity and specificity make them ideal for screening.

Such standalone tests include clock-drawing, the Mini-Mental Status Examination (MMSE), Montreal Cognitive Assessment (MoCA), the Brief Alzheimer Screen, and memory tests. These can include delayed recall and language fluency (e.g., generating words from a given category, like listing all the animals you can think of whose name begins with a particular letter, within sixty seconds).

Overall, such tests can distinguish normal cognition from dementia, although their ability to identify earlier states, such as MCI, from normal aging is unreliable.[229] Many can be successfully completed at home via computer and/or video with results comparable to face-to-face traditional testing.[230]

The Mini-Mental Status Examination (MMSE) is the most widely used screening tool for evaluating overall cognitive function. Best for detecting disturbances in memory and orientation,[72] the MMSE is highly sensitive for detecting MCI and AD.[89] The MMSE evaluates one's orientation to time and place; recent memory, attention, and concentration; the ability to perform skilled motor actions, and language. Easily administered in five to ten minutes, the MMSE is scored on a 30-point scale, with ≥25 classified as normal. Untreated patients with Alzheimer's disease decline at a rate of about two or three points each year.[206] (Note: If your doctor has ever had you recall the names of three objects after five minutes, spell backwards, or identify a pencil, you've taken the MMSE.)

The Montreal Cognitive Assessment (MoCA) evaluates orientation, memory, attention, language (naming), executive function and visuospatial function (clock drawing). In head-to-head studies with the MMSE, the MoCA appears more sensitive.[231]

The Blessed Dementia Scale is similar in content to the MMSE, but differs by including a second part completed by a caregiver. Caregivers list changes in the subject's everyday activities, personal habits, personality, interests, and drives.[206,231]

Quick tests (≤7 minutes): (1) The "Mini-Cog" (recall of three words and the clock-drawing task (drawing a clock face with numbers, and hands showing a specific time) is quicker and as accurate for dementia as the MMSE.[232] Recommended as a quick screen for the need for a specialty referral, it takes three minutes and has been formally recommended by the Alzheimer's Association because it can be completed within the time frame of a Medicare wellness visit.[233] (2) With the "Brief Alzheimer's Screening Test," the test-taker is asked to repeat three words immediately after hearing them, followed by two tasks that distract from those words. Finally, the person is asked to remember and recite the three words again.[234] (3)The "Six-Item Screen" consists of three-word recall plus three time-orientation questions: counting backwards from twenty, stating the months of the year in reverse and learning an address.[235] (4)The "Seven-Minute Screen" tests orientation (month, date, year, time); memory (sixteen items: four at a time); clock drawing; and verbal fluency (naming animals again). Published studies indicate sensitivity and specificity for dementia of greater than 90%.[236]

Accuracy and safety of single tests: The MMSE, MoCA, and Brief Alzheimer Screen standalone tests, delayed list-recall memory tests, and language fluency tests seem to be the most accurate, with sensitivities and specificities of approximately 0.90 or higher. These are all less accurate in distinguishing mild CATD (Clinical Alzheimer's-Type Dementia) from normal cognition, or distinguishing CATD from MCI. No studies of single tests reported harms.[229]

Longitudinal Testing Can Be More Revealing

Beginning five to eight years before the onset of dementia, decreasing accuracy when performing repeated neuropsychological tests, deterioration in activities of daily living, and increasing subjective concerns start to appear. When small trends in scores on individual components of a test battery are merged over repeated sessions, changes over time can expose subtle decline.[58] Reviewing such "composite scores" can reveal cognitive changes even in the preclinical stage.

Early diagnosis when AD is developing "silently" has significant implications. Finding effective early interventions for such a late-onset disorder could amount to prevention for some, and push decline later into the life span for others.[65]

Non-Traditional Measurements of Cognitive Decline

Language

Analysis of spontaneous (conversational) speech: (See also "Speech analysis by Artificial Intelligence" below). The spoken-language features of cognitive decline are mostly studied by analyzing transcribed spontaneous speech. Errors made by AD patients can include deteriorating fluency, increased pauses, progressively impaired naming, semantic errors (using category names like "my pet" instead of the target's name, "Rover"), and circumlocutory speech (excessively long descriptions or unnecessary details).[237]

Those of you who have had basic neurocognitive testing may remember the "cookie-theft picture." Here, you are asked to identify all the features and tell the story of a child falling from a stool while climbing to get a cookie while Mom dries a dish at an overflowing sink. Interestingly, it is the speech patterns one uses to describe that picture (as opposed to the ability to enumerate all of its content) that can identify early AD.[238,239]

Various quantifiable characteristics of spontaneous speech have been identified as reflecting the early stages of AD and are used to screen and monitor its progression. These include tempo (words per minute), complexity, pauses (frequency and length), numbers of unique words and conversational fillers, and the use of non-specific nouns over time.[237,238,240-245] A historical example confirming the presence of early dementia from analysis of spontaneous speech was a study of President Ronald Reagan's transcribed unscripted news conferences.[246]

Concerns for one's own speech can increase one's sensitivity to the speech patterns of others. Such awareness may prove useful, both in normal conversation and when you detect difficulties with spontaneous speech in others: especially your doctor, lawyer, senator, or accountant! Sometimes it does "take one to know one."

Increased pronoun use: The frequency of pronoun use in speech increases in the early phases of AD, interfering with both communication and understanding.[247] In a small study, the *spontaneous* speech of eleven patients with AD employed a greater ratio of pronouns to full noun phrases than the speech of nine healthy controls. These findings were thought to be due to impaired working memory, rather than difficulty with word-finding.[248]

The Pronoun Trap: Personal Observations

In speech: The increased tendency to overuse pronouns in everyday speech has rarely been studied. Only fifteen published papers on the topic were found in the National Library of Medicine database from 1985 to June, 2022! Yet, with aging, I find myself more frequently falling into this imprecise speech pattern.

It took a while to recognize the increased communication difficulties associated with dysfunctional pronoun substitutions. The pronoun trap occurs most frequently in conversations with my wife and is most likely secondary to our over fifty years of shared experiences. We both will occasionally fail to properly decode the pronouns that the other is using. One will start a sentence or resume a conversation with "he, she, they." That pronoun would be continuing a course of thought that the speaker had either just begun, silently, or had left behind in conversation a few minutes earlier. The other party will often then mentally attach a noun currently in mind, to that pronoun. At that point, the two sides of the conversation begin to diverge, eventually making little sense to either of us. Once we had it figured out, we would shake our heads, smile, say "pronouns!" out loud together, and then clarify the exchange.

With age, it seems to become progressively easier to swap a pronoun for a more specific proper noun. Regrettably, what often follows is making less and less sense while smoothly filling in the blanks. Although unconsciously substituting pronouns lowers the clarity and quality of conversation, it does not equate with "tip-of-the-tongue" (TOT) or word-finding difficulties. Those create noticeable hesitations in word flow, a disruption that can be perceived by others.

Writing: I also see similar pronoun substitutions in my writing. A first draft will often resemble careless spontaneous speech, with too many pronouns muddling communication. During revisions, I frequently find myself improving clarity by replacing pronouns with the proper noun to which I was referring.

I blame failing working memory for the Pronoun Trap. The proper noun referenced at the beginning of the paragraph or conversation is gone from recollection and replaced with a pronoun, resulting in a loss of clarity and accuracy.

Written Language: Techniques for diagnosing cognitive decline by reviewing a transcribed speech have also been successfully applied to the published works of authors who, like Agatha Christie, were subsequently diagnosed with dementia.[249-251]

Handwriting: "Agraphia" (a loss in the ability to communicate through writing) is one of the first signs of Alzheimer's disease. Writing gets shaky due to the loss of muscle control, confusion, and forgetfulness.[252,253]

Visuospatial, Sensory, and Motor Clues to Cognitive Decline

Visuospatial: Positive results from a digital Clock Drawing Test[254] were associated with amyloid and tau burden in clinically normal older adults.[255] Driving requires "functional visual acuity," the ability to operate a vehicle in response to visual information. Healthy elderly subjects with MCI were found to have a decrease in such visual abilities as orientation, attention, calculation, and recall. This, despite having no decrease in measured visual acuity.[256]

Handgrip strength (HGS): Diminished grip strength is considered the most reliable measure of muscle weakness. General weakness is associated with a wide range of health conditions, including AD. HGS asymmetry and weakness were associated with lower cognitive functioning in a national sample of over seventeen thousand aging Americans.[257,258]

Artificial Intelligence and Computer-Aided Assessments

Speech analysis by Artificial Intelligence (AI): Machine learning applied to transcribed doctor-patient conversations in a memory clinic correctly identified cognitive failings from neurodegenerative disease.[259] When asked, "Tell me everything you see going on" in the commonly employed "cookie-theft picture" (see "Analysis of spontaneous (conversational) speech," on page 109), AI distinguished AD patients from normal controls.[242] It took AI less than a ten-minute analysis of spontaneous speech to identify dementia "with accuracy comparable to existing diagnostic methods."[260] A mobile phone app has effectively differentiated among SCI, MCI and AD.[241]

Predictive algorithms, with or without AI, can also be diagnostic. The presence of eight personal risk factors accurately predicted the six-year risk of cognitive impairment in over ten thousand Chinese adults.[261] Findings from patients at memory clinics suggest that machine learning (artificial intelligence) could accurately forecast the occurrence of dementia within two years using only six variables: four from common neurocognitive tests, plus clinical judgments of decline and level of independence.[262]

Computerized cognitive assessments: The US Food and Drug Administration has approved the marketing of "CognICA, an artificial-intelligence-powered integrated cognitive assessment program to detect the early presence of dementia." This is a five-minute, computerized test that one can complete on an iPad.[263]

Buyer Beware! FDA approval for commercial distribution as a medical device may make it "available for purchase," but it does not validate consistency or accuracy. I question the scientific basis of the claim that CognICA provides a "sensitive and accurate measure of cognitive function," since I was unable to find a single publication mentioning that device when searching the National Institutes of Health (PubMed) database through April 2023.

Voice assistants: Research is ongoing to use voice-assistant systems (Alexa and others) for early detection of cognitive decline from dementia. This is seen as particularly beneficial for older adults living alone.[264]

"Alexa, how long before I finish this chapter?" Hey, developers, how about a personal AI that follows my conversations and beams the correct word from the tip of my tongue into my exchange?

Screening questionnaires

Informant-based questionnaires are a recent trend in screening for cognitive dysfunction. They ask a caregiver, friend or relative to answer questions about the patient's memory and other cognitive functions. Typically completed before an appointment or in the waiting room, the results can be made available to clinicians before evaluation. Such questionnaires may be preferable to other screening methods because: (1) they require no time from medical professionals; (2) there is no need for patient cooperation; (3) they can be accomplished via telephone, mail, or internet; and (4) they can be completed confidentially.[205]

Specific questionnaires include:

IQCODE (the Informant Questionnaire on Cognitive Decline in the Elderly): Sixteen items rate the degree of change in the patient's memory and intelligence over a ten-year period. It takes ten to fifteen minutes to administer and is as sensitive as the MMSE in identifying dementia (with an overall accuracy of 80–85%).[206]

The AD8 takes three minutes and can be completed by either an informant or the patient. Eight items are scored by identifying changes in cognitive abilities "over several years." Measures include judgment and the level of interest, repetition, learning new gadgets, financial tasks, remembering dates and appointments, and any daily problems with these.[265,266]

The score is simply the number of changed ("yes") items out of eight over time. A value ≥2 is felt to be highly suspicious for cognitive impairment and merits further evaluation for a definite diagnosis.[267]

Sensitivity and specificity for both are greater than 80%. While both the AD8 and IQCODE detect dementia in a community setting, the AD8 was more successful in detecting MCI.

The Alzheimer's Disease Caregiver Questionnaire (ADCQ) is an eighteen-item yes/no questionnaire that can be completed in five to ten minutes. It asks about multiple aspects of cognition, including memory, language, executive function, visuospatial and organized motor abilities. The ADCQ also assesses functional status, mood, and behavior, as well as for progression of symptoms. Validation studies have indicated nearly 90% accuracy in identifying patients who have symptoms of dementia suggestive of Alzheimer's disease.[206]

Stay tuned: More tests will be invented, studied, and used. Most will require years of longitudinal assessment to validate their ability to accurately indicate a progression to clinical AD.[58]

Risk Factors for Developing AD

The Definition and Evolution of Risk: The Science of Epidemiology

Risk is established by applying the tools of epidemiology,[268] "the study of how often diseases occur in different groups of people and why." A major feature of epidemiology's evolution has been an increase in its ability to determine the causes behind identified statistical associations.[269]

The nature of risk factors:[263] A risk factor is anything (environmental, habitual, acquired, or inherited) that increases a person's chances of developing a disease. Cigarette smoking (an acquired habit) is a well-known risk factor for lung cancer.

High blood pressure (an individual trait) is a risk for heart disease. It is important to distinguish between *causal* risk factors that directly underlie the biology of a disease vs. *predictive* risk factors used solely to identify those in jeopardy.

It is equally important to remember that, when dealing with percentages, the ability to predict the occurrence of clinical events in any single individual based on their risk-factor status is limited.[270] Not all smokers get cancer. Not all lung cancer patients smoked.

Risk factors are based on statistics. Their presence is simply counted in two otherwise similar groups: one with, and one without, the disease in question. Otherwise, the groups should be equivalent in age, sex distribution, and other biological, social, or environmental variables. If a factor is found more commonly in AD patients, the more likely it is that its presence can predict disease in others.

This type of study cannot assert causation, but rather identifies and quantifies statistical associations. Age, for example, a risk factor common to many conditions, does not cause all the maladies with which it is negatively associated.

Risk factors are determined from large and longitudinal epidemiological studies. Their results often drive health standards and recommendations, most commonly expressed as what *not* to do to lower one's likelihood of developing a disease. Think smoking.

Risk factors are continually reevaluated as large groups are reassessed over time, and relationships between outcomes and various risk factors are clarified. Recommendations can change when the next large study comes out. Statistical associations will continue to be discovered and fall in and out of favor. For instance, "good cholesterol" used to be an oxymoron!

Focusing on the inevitable inconsistencies in such data can lead one to ignore beneficial lifestyle modifications. At some point, there will likely be a new study to the contrary. Awareness of risk factors has its greatest value in possibilities for primary and secondary prevention by risk factor modification. Most prominently, risk-factor modification has been key to both preventing and managing cardiovascular disease.

Risk factors for AD can be categorized as those that are modifiable (and often lifestyle-related) and those that are not.

One example of the inevitable changes that occur in the science of assigning risk hit particularly close to home. In a study that I eagerly took to heart, afternoon napping in a group of elderly Chinese was associated with better cognitive function.[271] In subsequent work—which was very disturbing to me—napping for an hour came with a 29% increase in AD mortality when compared with no nap.[272,273] However—conflict resolved! Worrying about the fatal downside of napping now keeps me awake. Sometimes you just can't win.

Unmodifiable Risk Factors for AD

Age: We're living longer. The risk of developing dementia varies with age[274], particularly after seventy. Age also plays an indirect role via the contribution of age-associated comorbidities.[58]

Sex: The fact that more women than men develop AD initially led to the conclusion that females have an increased risk.[65] Confounding the sex difference is the fact that, on average, women live longer than men, reinforcing older age as the number one AD risk. Most attempts to identify the actual risk of developing dementia for men and women of the *same age* have failed to find any significant difference between the sexes.[117] However, in middle-aged women, hormonal risk factors, particularly menopause, do predict AD, suggesting that a primary window of opportunity for AD prevention in women is early in the endocrine aging process.[275]

Genetics: "Approximately 70% of the risk of developing AD can be attributed to genetics."[167] (See "The Genetic Basis of AD," page 81.)

> This book is primarily aimed at the millions of us aging into our memory concerns. Understanding the genetics of AD and its novel language is equally important to the millions of our relatives.

Any *family history* of AD increases one's risk of AD by three to four times. *Forty-one percent of first-degree relatives (parents, siblings or children) will develop the disease by the ninth decade of life.*[7] First-degree relatives of late-onset AD patients have a two-to-three-fold increased AD risk, and will often do so at a similar age as their family member. Fortunately, the three dominant causative genes leading to early-onset AD are rare. Found in fewer than 450 families, they likely account for half of the cases of AD occurring before age sixty.

Twin studies have classically been used to assess if increased risk in families is due to genetic factors. Identical (monozygotic) twins, who share all their genes, show concordance, meaning both will have (or lack) the same genetic traits, like eye color. Fraternal (dizygotic) twins are just like ordinary siblings who share only half their genes. Even monozygotic twins do not uniformly come to share an AD diagnosis, and, when they do, their age of onset may differ by 10 or more years.[65]

APOE: "Alleles" are alternate versions of a gene that occur at a particular location. For example, imagine a hair-color gene hanging out in your DNA, maybe squashed between Uncle Harry's buck teeth and Grandma's high cholesterol. Your DNA has two inherited hair-color alleles attached to your hair-color gene—one from each parent. If the two alleles are the same, you are homozygous for that gene.

Apolipoprotein E is a protein that our cells produce in one of three forms (E2, E3, and E4). Which protein version we manufacture depends upon and identifies which of these three possible alleles we inherited from our parents. There is a lot of discussion around testing for APOE4. The E4 allele of apolipoprotein E (APOE) is the strongest genetic risk factor for the common (late-onset) form of AD.[276] APOE is a *susceptibility* gene controlling the likelihood of developing AD without actually causing the disease. APOE4 is present in 40%–60% of AD cases,[7,65] and, along with its two other inherited versions (alleles 2, and 3), also impacts the risk for cardiovascular disease.

The most common genotype (APOE3) is considered neutral concerning AD risk,[277] while APOE2 actually decreases risks for both AD and cardiovascular disease. However, those individuals bearing one or two copies of APOE4 exhibit a higher risk of developing AD (as well as cardiovascular disease and decreased longevity) when compared to noncarriers. It was the presence of APOE4 in biomarker-positive patients that helped identify, quantify, and validate the association of this genetic carrier state with markers of AD.[54,78-82] The APOE4 allele acts principally by modifying the main age for AD onset, estimated at sixty-eight years in E-4 homozygotes, seventy-six years in E-4 heterozygotes, and eighty-four years in noncarriers.[58] APOE4 carriers with self-reported cognitive concerns (SCD, chapter 2) experience cognitive decline more rapidly than noncarriers.[75-77] With or without cognitive symptoms, the prevalence of amyloid is two to three times higher in APOE4 carriers than in noncarriers, an effect that appears to be stronger in women and in Caucasians, which may relate to those groups' lower risk of cardiovascular disease.[65]

In addition to APOE, over forty risk gene variations involved in lipid metabolism, the inflammatory response, and certain cell functions have also been identified in AD. Most are common, with limited effects.[58,171]

In summary, while increasing the risk, "Inheritance of an APOE4 allele neither defines the presence of Alzheimer's pathologic change or AD nor indicates any particular stage of the disease."[133]

Genetic syndromes with increased AD risk: Down syndrome is a well-established genetic risk factor for AD.[278,279] Increased life expectancy has led to an associated increase in age-related conditions, especially AD, the main medical problem and leading cause of death in this population. Amyloid plaques and tau neurofibrillary tangles are virtually universal by age forty, and the lifetime risk of developing dementia is over 90%.[280]

Also associated with AD are Inflammatory Bowel Disease[281] and Attention-Deficit/Hyperactivity Disorder (ADHD). In a very large cohort of families of ADHD patients, relatives across generations (parents, grandparents, uncles/aunts) had an increased probability of a diagnosis of AD, with parents having the greatest risk.[282]

Genetic syndromes with *decreased* AD risk are being identified as well.[283]

The role of genetic testing in the evaluation of AD:[65] (See also above.) In assessing risk, be sure not to confuse genes with biomarkers. Biomarkers are the "fingerprints" of the disease itself, proof of its existence in the body. However, the existence of a susceptibility gene does not signal the presence of amyloid or tau. Also, unlike biomarkers, they have no role in diagnosis or staging. Except for the very rare patient with familial (early onset) AD, genetic variations do not cause AD.

Genes are responsible for the transfer of traits and susceptibilities from one generation to the next. Sometimes these result in the emergence of specific diseases, and sometimes they interact with one's behavior and environment to trigger the expression of other traits. As with all other risk factors, genomic testing provides a measure of probability. *Roughly 50% of those who develop sporadic AD do not possess the E4 allele*, clearly indicating that other factors are involved.[7]

Patients with a family member with dementia often ask whether they should test for their own risk of AD. Those with an autosomal dominant family history (early-onset Alzheimer's disease) who are concerned about symptoms are best served by seeking genetic counseling. Of the three dominant early-onset AD genes, however, there is presently only a commercial test for one. Tests for the others only exist in research settings. Those without a family autosomal dominant pattern can be told that there is a modestly increased risk of AD in first-degree relatives (parent, sibling, or child) and that the age of onset tends to be similar.

The current advice is: "Genetic testing for APOE can be used as an adjunct to diagnosis, but it contributes minimally. It is not recommended for the assessment of future risk because it lacks sufficient predictive value at the individual level. Many normal elderly carry an APOE4 allele, and many AD patients do not."[65]

Potentially Modifiable Risk Factors—Action Could Slow or Prevent AD

The World Health Organization has taken the position that "while age is the strongest known risk factor for cognitive decline, dementia is not a natural or inevitable consequence of aging. Aging without dementia is achievable."[180]

For this, we turn to "primary prevention"—those measures aimed at a susceptible population or healthy individuals to prevent a disease from ever occurring. Primary prevention involves lessening the potential impact of an identified risk factor. It is the existence of potentially modifiable risk factors that makes slowing the onset or progression or even *avoiding* dementia, possible.[180] Recommended risk-reduction activities are simple to follow, and also benefit one's overall health and well-being.[65]

There are many modifiable lifestyle-related risk factors associated with the development of cognitive impairment and dementia. (See table 2.)[115,180,284] In addition to the validation of their presence by one or more scientific studies, the twelve risk factors specifically identified in the table by asterisks were strongly endorsed by the interdisciplinary, international group of experts authoring the 2020 report of the Lancet Commission on Dementia Prevention, Intervention, and Care.[115]

To support their conclusions, these experts attributed recently observed declines in the age-specific incidence of dementia in many countries to lifestyle changes and improvements in education, nutrition, and health care. They concluded that *"modifying at least these 12 risk factors might prevent or delay up to 40% of dementias."* The National Institute on Aging (NIA) provides a similar to-do list of preventive steps for cognitive health: "Cognitive Health and Older Adults."[285]

The connection of dementia cases in the US with potentially modifiable risk factors is especially strong for Black and Hispanic individuals.[286]

Table 2: Potentially Modifiable AD Risk Factors

Multiple lifestyle-related risk factors are related to the development of cognitive impairment and dementia. Modifying the twelve starred (*) risk factors is believed to potentially prevent or delay up to 40% of dementias.[115]	
Table 2.1 - Lifestyle Factors with Increased Dementia Risk	
Lifestyle Risk Factor	**Comment**
Physical Inactivity	Low to moderate levels of physical activity in later life significantly reduce the risk for age-related dementia.[287,288]
Smoking	
Obesity	

2.1 (Continued)

Excessive Alcohol Consumption	"Alcohol-induced loss of consciousness is a long-term risk factor for dementia among both heavy and moderate drinkers."[289]
Cognitive Inactivity	
Unhealthy Diets	Greater intake of ultra-processed foods was associated with cognitive decline and dementia among adults, while unprocessed or minimally processed foods lowered dementia risk.[290,291]
Long-term Cannabis Use	Weed smokers experienced cognitive deficits and smaller hippocampal brain volume in midlife.[292]
Sleep Duration	Both short *and* long sleep durations were associated with worse outcomes for older adults, including increases in amyloid burden, depressive symptoms, body mass index, and cognitive decline.[293] The latest data puts the sleep duration "sweet spot" at around seven hours.[294]

Table 2.2 - Medical Conditions with Increased Dementia Risk	
Medical Risk Factor	**Comment**
Hypertension[295]	Treatment of hypertension decreases AD brain findings,[296] and the risk of subsequent dementia.[297]
Diabetes[167]	
Depression[167]	
Traumatic Brain Injury (TBI)	Any history of severe head trauma (with loss of consciousness) or any moderate-to-severe TBI increases the risk of subsequent Alzheimer's disease.[298]
Hearing impairment[13,299,300]	Hearing loss is found in 8% of dementia cases and is linked to an increased risk of MCI and accelerated cognitive decline. *Hearing aid users were less likely to develop MCI*

2.2 (Continued)

	and all-cause dementia compared to those not using hearing aids.[301,302] *[Show this to Mom or Dad when they won't wear their hearing aids!]*
Vision Impairment[13]	This is a risk factor for accelerated cognitive decline and developing dementia.[115] An estimated 90% of vision loss is preventable or has yet to be treated.[303]
Hypercholesterolemia	
Cerebrovascular Diseases	
Atherosclerosis	
Atrial Fibrillation	
COVID-19 Infection	Elderly patients were at significantly increased risk for a new diagnosis of Alzheimer's disease within one year post-COVID diagnosis, particularly women, or age eighty-five and over.[304]
Herpes Zoster (Shingles)	Varicella zoster virus (VZV) has been implicated in Alzheimer's disease, and vaccination against shingles, caused by VZV, has been found to decrease the risk of AD/dementia.[305]
Positional variability in systolic blood pressure	Low blood pressure when standing.[306]
Sleep-disordered breathing[65,307]	
Accumulated metabolic byproducts of various foods.[308]	
Distressing dreams	Bad dreams predict cognitive decline and all-causes of dementia in middle-aged and older men without preexisting cognitive impairment.[309]

2.2 (Continued)

ICU hospitalization	ICU hospitalization was associated with double the risk of dementia in community-based older adults compared to those who did not experience ICU hospitalization.[310]
Delirium during a hospitalization	This phenomenon was significantly associated with long-term cognitive decline in both surgical and nonsurgical patients.[311]

Table 2.3 - Social/Environmental (S&E) Factors with Increased Dementia Risk	
S&E Risk Factor	**Comment**
Less education	
Social isolation	
Air pollution	
Noise pollution	Long-term exposure to residential transportation noise increased the risk of all-cause dementia, especially Alzheimer's disease.[312]
Widowhood[313]	

References:

a. Risk Reduction of Cognitive Decline and Dementia: WHO Guidelines (2019)[180]

b. Livingston, G., et al., *Dementia Prevention, Intervention, and Care: 2020 Report of the Lancet Commission*. Lancet, 2020. 396(10248): p. 413-446.[115]

c. Baumgart, M., et al. (2015). "Summary of the evidence on modifiable risk factors for cognitive decline and dementia: A population-based perspective." *Alzheimers Dement* 11(6): 718-726.[284]

d. "Preventing Cognitive Decline and Dementia: A Way Forward, National Academies of of of Sciences, Engineering, and Medicine (2017).[183]

e. Kane, R. L., et al. (2017). "Interventions to Prevent Age-Related Cognitive Decline, Mild Cognitive Impairment, and Clinical Alzheimer's-Type Dementia." (AHRQ, Rockville, MD)[182]

Why haven't we, the public, heard of AD prevention from these major government-funded academic sources? The same sort of measures they already actively promote to unclog our arteries, bring down our blood sugars, mellow our depression, or curb our self-destructive habits should merit similar emphasis.

In 2017, seemingly all the US experts (convened by both the National Academies of Sciences and the Agency for Healthcare Research and Quality) combined to review dementia prevention (see references d. and e. in table 2.3[183,182]).

The conclusion of the National Academies' 180-page effort (Reference d.) was disappointing:

"There is insufficient high-strength experimental evidence to justify a public health information campaign, per se, that would encourage the adoption of specific interventions to prevent these conditions."[183]

Really??? In my opinion, the overall benefits of reasonable wellness approaches are already accepted as appropriate for the general public. If nearly nine hundred pages of scholarly analysis of data from 1906 to 2017 yielded only "encouraging although inconclusive evidence," we have a long way to go. Personally, I would rather have the information and judge for myself, and that is why I'm passing it on to you.

Also, if "encouraging although inconclusive" is the highest degree of certainty that can be achieved from volumes of expert-published, peer-reviewed scientific evidence, then relying on advertisements, testimonials, doubtful "clinical studies," or celebrity endorsements seems particularly foolish.

Due diligence by patients, families, and physicians requires skepticism and risk/benefit analysis before accepting and embarking on any strategy recommended for prevention, delay, or treatment.

Why not try as many helpful suggestions as you can? Just stick with those that your doctor can verify as not harmful and potentially beneficial. A worthwhile formula to select options for modifying any health risk factors is: (1) Be sure the recommendation has been proven to be beneficial. (2) Be sure it has the potential to support your cognitive health.

(1) +(2) = WIN+WIN

Targeting Some Risks Has Been Effective

An early randomized controlled trial in elders at risk of dementia demonstrated that a two-year intervention program of nutritional guidance, exercise, cognitive training, social stimulation, and management of vascular and metabolic risk factors could actually improve or maintain cognitive functioning.[314] Other studies found that a Mediterranean diet and programs of physical exercise were associated with decreased brain AD-burden among cognitively intact individuals.[58]

In a UK study of over seventy-eight thousand adults aged 40–79 followed for a median of seven years, *walking* 9,826 steps per day was associated with a 49% lower risk of all-cause dementia, with roughly half that benefit from 3,826 steps daily.[315]

A greater long-term intake of vegetables and fruits is associated with maintaining cognitive function later in life, lowering the incidence of subjective cognitive decline.[60] A 2020 review and meta-analysis of 396 studies of risk factor modification "identified a total of 21 evidence-based suggestions . . . to pre-vent AD." Nearly two-thirds of these targeted vascular risk fac-tors and lifestyle.[316]

Score yourself! Dhana, et al. created a lifestyle scoring system ranging from 0–5, with one point for each of five positive lifestyle choices: non-smoking, weekly moderate/vigorous-intensity phys-ical activity, light to moderate alcohol consumption, high-qual-ity Mediterranean-DASH diet, and engagement in late-life cognitive activities. For the 2,765 elderly subjects (mostly over seventy and initially without dementia) studied over a median of six years, higher scores were "associated with a substantially lower risk of Alzheimer's dementia." Compared to participants with zero to one healthy lifestyle factors, the risk of Alzheimer dementia was 37% lower in those with two to three healthy life-style factors and 60% lower in those with four to five.[317]

"Encouraging Although Inconclusive Evidence" for Reducing Risk of MCI or AD

These come from the large 2017 National Academies Report[183] or more recent single studies awaiting replication, validation, and wider acceptance by such agencies.

Being **physically active** does delay or slow Age-Related Cognitive Decline (ARCD),[182] but is "without sufficient evidence to identify an effect on MCI or CATD ("Clinical Alzheimer's-Type Dementia")."[183] Physical exercise coupled with greater lifetime cognitive activity has been associated with lower brain beta-amy-loid burden and fewer cerebrovascular AD lesions.[58] Among par-ticipants with both high and low total tau concentrations, physical activity was associated with slower cognitive decline.[287]

Avoid **"Repetitive Negative Thinking"** (**RNT**): RNT, also termed "perseverative cognition" is described as "excessive and repetitive thinking about current concerns, problems, past experiences, or worries about the future." RNT is rumination that frequently accompanies psychiatric diagnoses that are also risk factors for AD. These include depression, anxiety, PTSD, and substance use disorder. Measurable and potentially modifiable, RNT is associated with the presence of AD markers in cognitively intact older adults. Higher levels of RNT were coupled with more rapid decline in global memory and cognition over forty-eight months, as well as higher levels of tau in the brain.[318,319]

Cognitive training: see non-drug (behavioral) interventions later in this chapter.

Improved blood pressure (BP) control: Since better control of hypertension can reduce stroke incidence and mortality from cerebrovascular disease, it could very plausibly moderate AD via the same mechanism. While the overall health benefits of maintaining optimal BP are undeniable, randomized controlled studies do not offer strong support for antihypertension treatment to delay or slow ARCD, MCI, or Alzheimer's-type dementia. Research is hindered by the ethical difficulties of including a control group in whom hypertension is not treated to directly test the beneficial effects of blood pressure management on cognition. One more recent study found that the use of anti-hypertensive medications was associated with a lower likelihood of most neurodegenerative diseases, with diuretics the class most strongly associated with this decrease.[320]

Diet: The MIND diet is a hybrid of the Mediterranean diet and the Dietary Approaches to Stop Hypertension (DASH) diet. It is reported to slow cognitive decline in older adults and reduce the risk of AD.[321] "Drinking coffee and tea separately or in combination were associated with lower risks of stroke and dementia."[322]

Alcohol: "Low to moderate" amounts of alcohol are supported for risk reduction, along with reducing alcohol consumption from a heavy to a moderate level, and even the initiation of mild alcohol consumption. Alcohol "dosage" had a "U-shaped association with all cognitive function domains for all participants, with an optimal dose of 10 to 14 drinks per week."[323,324]

Watching TV did not affect multiple cognitive domains in older adult residents of São Paulo, Brazil.[325] More than three and a half hours a day is associated with a dose-related decline in verbal memory over the following six years.[326]

Sleep duration: There is an inverted U-shaped association between sleep duration and overall cognitive decline; i.e., avoid too much or too little. Go for the "sweet spot." Short sleep duration in midlife has an increased risk of late-onset dementia.[327] Looking at data from almost five hundred thousand European (i.e., Caucasian) adults, Li, et al. concluded that *seven hours of sleep per night is optimal* for mental health, well-being, and cognitive performance for people in their late thirties to early seventies.[273] Insufficient ($\leq$ 4 hours per night) or excessive ($\geq$ 10 hours) sleep times led to worse cognitive decline,[328,329] as well as greater beta-amyloid burden, more depressive symptoms, and higher body mass index.[293]

Other work identifies an optimal sleep time between four and a half and six and a half hours per night that stabilized cognitive function in a longitudinal study. Older adults with sleep durations outside that range reported significant cognitive decline over the same period.[330]

Prevention of Traumatic Brain Injury (TBI): Repeated TBIs in athletes (boxers and football players have been most extensively studied) both increases AD risk and can cause Chronic Traumatic Encephalopathy (CTE). Like AD in its earlier days, CTE can, so far, only be diagnosed at autopsy.[298,331]

Sports teams are beginning to make changes that reflect increasing concern for CTE and the incidence of TBI-associated AD. Brain-specific blood-based protein biomarkers have recently been approved by the FDA to identify TBI/concussion, and will hopefully result in increased risk-awareness for those engaging in contact sports.[332] Alas, it will be a long time before the effects of such improvements will be felt by those who experience TBI.

Parents of wannabe football players will hopefully
come to their senses
before their children lose theirs.

"Mamas, don't let your babies grow up
to be [Dallas] cowboys"
(after Waylon Jennings & Willie Nelson, 1978)

The Bottom Line on Possibly Modifiable Risk Factors

There is a wide span of "evidence" when it comes to possible ways to modify risk factors. Published reviews of such possibilities nearly always include the caveat, "more studies are needed." Some of us may choose to adopt the results of appealing, but preliminary, studies and experiment on ourselves. Because Alzheimer's is such a complex disease with great variability in onset, progression, and outcome, understand this:

Any preventive effort one person might undertake is basically a coin-flip experiment with only one subject.

With no control group for comparison, there is no way to exclude the effects of chance, genetics, or some other unmeasured or unmeasurable variable. No matter how strong one's impression of benefit might be, *no individual will ever know* if that daily Brussels sprout, jellyfish parfait, celebrity-endorsed supplement, brisk walk, or crossword puzzle has had any real impact on the trajectory of their cognitive aging.

On the other hand, making healthy lifestyle modifications that, in general, will maximize your overall quality of life *is* worth a try. Any low-risk effort to postpone the onset of MCI or delay progression to dementia can potentially alter the disease trajectory by improving life expectancy and possibly limiting time spent in the end-stages of AD and in nursing home settings. Even modest delays in the onset of MCI can have beneficial outcomes.[196]

Primary Prevention That Can Inhibit AD Development

"One More Question, Doc"?

Dr. Ivan Koychev, an Alzheimer's researcher, has said that he hears this frequently: "How can I avoid getting Alzheimer's?" This "one more question" is a frequent parting query from the son or daughter of a patient recently diagnosed with dementia. It is brought up just as they are about to leave—almost as an afterthought."[223] Here are some honest answers:

Resilience

While much research focuses on risk factors for developing dementia, the interaction between such external influences and one's personal brain development is far from direct. Unique variations exist among individuals in their "resilience," a characteristic that incorporates both *resistance* to expected age-related brain changes and *protection* from the toxicity of accumulating amyloid and tau proteins. Identified "resilient" people have avoided dementia despite extreme old age, even though some possessed brains indistinguishable from their peers with Alzheimer's disease! Of 276 autopsy cases, all of which had significant levels of AD pathology, 25% were characterized as "resilient." They had never received a clinical diagnosis of dementia and had scored ≥86 out of 100 on a Cognitive Abilities Screening Instrument within the two years before their death.[333] As many as 70% of cognitively unimpaired older adults have some level of AD pathology present in the brain at death,[171] while nearly half of centenarians with dementia lacked sufficient brain pathology to explain their cognitive symptoms. Such inconsistencies suggest that individual compensatory mechanisms may help some seniors escape AD, even in extreme old age, and often despite disease-defining anatomical changes.[334] In the context of brain health, resilience is not a completely built-in quality, nor does being resilient mean never having been vulnerable in the first place. Rather, the brain has so-called counter-regulatory mechanisms that build resilience to combat negative change.[335] Identifying genetic and other factors promoting resilience among amyloid-positive individuals offers targets for clinical intervention and has inspired the development of experimental drugs.[194,195]

Inherited resilience factors: Newer analyses have identified "genes of resilience" that modify the relationship between the extent of baseline amyloid deposition and the degree of cognitive change. Such findings may explain those long preclinical periods in which some people avoid memory loss and other symptoms of AD even as they develop the brain signatures of the disease,[194] demonstrating "better cognitive performance than they should have, given how much amyloid was in their brains."[195] Inactivation of one specific gene (CD33) appears to confer protection against AD, by reducing amyloid levels and associated plaque burden.[336]

Support for the concept of genetic resilience comes from the study of one surprisingly lucky patient born with a rare mutation that usually results in high brain amyloid and very early AD (age forties to fifties). This individual, however, avoided cognitive impairment until her seventies, three decades after her expected age of clinical onset. She was "protected" against her rare amyloid-generating gene by an equally rare APOE3 gene mutation, the study of which could be beneficial for promoting resilience.[277,337]

AGE => AD is not inevitable.

Acquired Protection through "Cognitive Reserve"

Along with inherent characteristics like resilience, some acquired protective factors and compensatory mechanisms may help protect against AD.

Who: Cognitive reserve (CR) is identified in individuals with significant educational and occupational achievements and engagement in leisure and social activities.

What: "Common surrogates for CR include years of schooling, job complexity, vocabulary level, literacy, and integrity of social networks."[338] Each of these factors has been shown to modulate the degree of AD detected via measurements of *in vivo* biomarkers. In observational studies, examples of CR have been linked to more successful aging and decreased risk of dementia.[58,117,339] For example, compared with those with less education, persons with the highest levels of education had a 40% decreased risk of Alzheimer's disease.[99] Half of autopsied individuals identified as "resilient" had a college degree, compared with 32% for "non-resilient."[333]

Woo-Hoo! I went to 23rd grade!

How: Interference with connections between distant brain regions is a feature of AD. CR is attributed to *acquired backup brain circuitry*, providing increased neural connections to buffer the effects of losing neurons and synapses to AD. More years of learning promote denser circuitry. The assumption is that if the original path is lost to Alzheimer's, then the brain can activate the backups. Thus, brains with greater cognitive reserve can lose more synapses and neurons to AD without effect: i.e., although there is the same amount of amyloid, there is less cognitive decline.[195,339-341]

Examples of activities generating Cognitive Reserve include:

(1) The nature of one's work: In a study of 107,896 participants, the risk of dementia in old age was lower in individuals with cognitively stimulating jobs than in those with non-stimulating jobs. This finding persisted with adjustments for education and established dementia risk factors. Job-related cognitive stimulation was also associated with lower levels of some plasma proteins believed to increase dementia risk.[342]

(2) Early-Life Cognitive Enrichment (ELCE): Oveisgharan et al. studied the brains of elderly subjects who had previously detailed the "Early-Life Cognitive Enrichment" they had experienced by ages six, eight, twelve, and eighteen. ELCE included socioeconomic status, parents' education, number of siblings, cognitive resources in the home (like a newspaper subscription, encyclopedia or atlas), reading and being read to, and early foreign language instruction. ELCE was associated with better late-life cognitive health, in part through fewer AD pathological changes.[343] Notably, these effects were independent of late-life socioeconomic status and late-life reports of cognitive activity, suggesting the benefits of early cognitive enrichment go beyond long-term changes in lifestyle or behavior.[344]

Bravo for preschool and at-home enrichment programs! These can potentially extend their benefits a lifetime beyond their stated purpose of promoting "school readiness of infants, toddlers, and preschool-aged children." They can help prevent or lessen the impact of dementia. Junior, do your homework! You'll thank me (much) later.

A caution: Dr. Daniel Gibbs, an academic neurologist who carefully chronicles his own developing Alzheimer's disease, made the following [edited] observations on cognitive reserve. They provide me with little comfort.

> Over the last two years, I've been very engaged intellectually in writing and reading research in the literature. I think that probably is slowing the progression of my disease. There is this concept of cognitive reserve. People who have more schooling tend to have less cognitive problems for the same degree of neuropathology in the brain. But *at a certain point, in their disease, they fall off the cliff* [emphasis added]. So, someone with high cognitive reserve does pretty well for a number of years, and then all of a sudden, they don't. And they can go into the later stages of Alzheimer disease very rapidly. Whereas somebody with a lesser cognitive reserve has a more constant slope of their deterioration over many, many years.[111]

I am someone whose identity has been defined by my level of education, my "cognitive reserve." Previously employed mainly to dumbfound elementary-school kids with the fact that I finally got my first job after completing <u>23rd grade</u>, I now, for the first time, find myself anxious about the future risks from all of that schooling.

Secondary Prevention: Slowing or Stopping AD

Options Available

Biomarkers can identify those at risk. Predictive biomarkers can detect the brain changes of AD decades before the onset of symptoms. They offer a wide window of opportunity for risk-factor modification to prevent or delay the onset of cognitive decline.[65,183]

Risk-reduction lifestyle interventions are under study for those with subjective cognitive decline (SCD) and mild cognitive impairment (MCI). In a randomized trial, SCD and MCI subjects completed online sessions promoting behaviors that reduce dementia risk. These include the Mediterranean Diet, physical activity, and cognitive engagement. Experimental subjects also had active lifestyle training (with a dietitian and exercise physiologist) and had completed brain training. *The active interventions both significantly decreased exposure to AD risk factors, and improved cognition in those experiencing cognitive decline.*[345,346] While the volume of research in this area continues to grow, anyone, at any age, can begin modifying their risk factors—today!

Managing diabetes: Treating Type II diabetes with Dipeptidyl Peptidase-4 Inhibitors (Gliptins) reduced amyloid burden in diabetic patients with AD-related cognitive impairment.[347]

Treating high blood pressure: Pooled individual data from more than twenty-eight thousand patients in five clinical trials supported the benefits of antihypertensive treatment in late midlife to later life in lowering the risk of dementia.[297]

"Differential Diagnosis": What Else Could It Be?

Dementia? or Not Dementia?

When memory issues begin to surface, this is the number one question, the reason for all the clock drawing and identifying common objects that your doctors (should) repeat yearly. Patients with dementia from any cause also suffer from: (1) substantial decline in one or more cognitive functions, including complex attention, executive function, learning and memory, language, or perceptual, motor, or social skills; (2) loss of independence in everyday activities of daily living.

Identifying the origin of the dementia syndrome. As with nearly every medical disorder, the clinical findings of dementia come with a list of possible causes that need to be "ruled out." Not all dementia patients have Alzheimer's disease. Other conditions should be carefully considered by an expert. Some causes on the list may be inherited, while others may respond to specific treatments or result in far different prognoses.[48]

The Neural Degenerative Dementias

Number one is Alzheimer's disease. Nearly 75% of all dementing illnesses in those over sixty-five are due at least in part to Alzheimer's. Therefore, most evaluations of cognitively impaired adults start with AD as a working hypothesis, while also seeking other common causes of cognitive impairment.[124]

Lewy Body Dementia is the next most common of the neurodegenerative dementias. While accumulation of beta-amyloid and tau in the brain cause AD, widespread deposits of a different abnormal protein form "Lewy bodies" inside brain cells. These interfere with chemical transmissions necessary for normal memory, learning, mood, and sleep. Cognition may fluctuate throughout the day. Parkinson's disease, which has its own associated dementia syndrome, can also be complicated by Lewy body dementia.[348]

Frontotemporal Dementia (FTD, or Frontotemporal Lobar Degeneration) results from shrinkage of the frontal and temporal lobes of the brain that control personality, behavior, and language.[349] The most publicly diagnosed is actor Bruce Willis. FTD is the most common form of dementia in people younger than age sixty.[350]

LATE (Limbic-predominant Age-related TDP-43 Encephalopathy) is caused by the buildup of a fourth abnormal protein in specific brain structures. It is commonly observed in subjects over eighty years old and clinically mimics Alzheimer's disease. LATE is being recognized more frequently, often coexisting and interacting with AD to accelerate cognitive decline.[351-353]

Less common neurodegenerative dementias comprise about 5% of the total dementia population[65,205] and include:

Chronic traumatic encephalopathy (CTE): CTE is a largely preventable degenerative dementia resulting from repeated bouts of traumatic brain injury (TBI). Even mild injuries from repetitive head trauma, often without concussion, increase the risk for CTE. A *single* moderate-to-severe TBI can also increase the risk of subsequent Alzheimer's disease.[298]

Progressive dysexecutive syndrome due to Alzheimer's disease is a newly described subtype of AD that affects organizing, planning, and other executive functions and strikes patients as early as in their forties;[354]

Others: Corticobasal degeneration; Creutzfeldt–Jakob disease; multiple sclerosis; normal pressure hydrocephalus; Parkinson's disease (which can occur with and without dementia); primary age-related tauopathy; primary progressive aphasia; and progressive supranuclear palsy. Combined with vascular dementia (below), neurodegenerative diseases account for up to 95% of all dementias in the elderly.[124]

Vascular Dementia

Like stroke, vascular dementia (also known as "multi-infarct dementia") is a result of aging and those conditions that promote hardening of the arteries (atherosclerosis). These include hypertension, elevated cholesterol, smoking, diabetes, etc. Vascular dementia is the second most common cause of cognitive loss and dementia overall, behind Alzheimer's disease. It is estimated to account for approximately a third of all dementia cases.[47]

Health Conditions That Can Mimic Dementia

The clinical syndrome of dementia can arise from medical conditions affecting memory and cognition. Although fewer than 15% of new dementia cases are reversible, it is important to consider and eliminate these less common—but potentially modifiable—causes as early as possible. Providers should perform a complete evaluation to rule out infectious disease and other causes as reasons for memory lapses and difficulty in focusing. They may also consider a psychiatric assessment to rule out depression, a common cause for lethargy and disorientation in the elderly.[147]

Post-COVID "brain fog": As part of the "long COVID" complex, there is growing recognition of persistent neurocognitive symptoms ("brain fog") that follow COVID-19 infections (including those not requiring hospitalization), that can be mistaken for cognitive decline.[355-357] Similar post-COVID–era symptoms that are unrelated to COVID-19 infection are attributable to the other unique secondary stressors of 2020–22 (lockdown, uncertainty, personal and family illness, etc.).[358]

Postoperative cognitive decline: Associated with anesthesia and surgery in older patients, postoperative cognitive dysfunction is a prolonged state of impairment that predominantly affects higher-level cognitive skills and memory.[359]

Medications and drug interactions[285]: Up to one-third of cases of memory complaints and cognitive dysfunction may be caused by medications. Much more common in the elderly, cognitive side effects are seen with multiple classes of medications, including many available over the counter. Polypharmacy and associated drug-drug interactions are common in this group. Any drug is suspect if its first prescription and the onset of symptoms are temporally related.[65]

Drugs that can harm older adults' cognition include: sedatives, opioids, corticosteroids, antihistamines for allergy relief, medicines for anxiety and depression, sleep aids, antipsychotics, muscle relaxants, some drugs for treating urinary incontinence, and medications for relief of cramps in the stomach, intestines, and bladder ("anticholinergics").[65,285]

Other identified medical causes of cognitive symptoms (many quite rare) include:[24,32,54,360,361]

- Infections of the brain (including HIV, neurosyphilis, and Lyme disease)
- Cancers of the brain itself or metastatic from other sources
- Some forms of seizures
- Inflammatory disorders such as vasculitis and thyroiditis
- Metabolic and endocrine diseases including diabetes, thyroid disease, and adrenal gland dysfunction
- Acute trauma with bleeding into the brain or surrounding spaces
- Organ failure: e.g., kidney, liver
- Dehydration
- Nutritional, vitamin, or enzyme deficiencies (like vitamin B-12)
- Environmental toxins
- Alcoholism and other substance use disorders
- Hydrocephalus

Behavioral and Psychiatric Conditions Can Mimic or Predict Dementia or Pre-Dementia Syndromes

Delirium is a common life-threatening *medical* emergency often confused with dementia. Delirium is generally more sudden in onset and observed after surgery, intoxication, or withdrawal in those with substance use disorder, and in patients with critical illnesses such as sepsis, respiratory failure, and cardiogenic shock. Delirium is marked by an acute onset or fluctuating course, inattention, and either disorganized thought (memory, language, and orientation difficulties) or an altered level of consciousness. Delirium can mimic dementia and be associated with long-term cognitive decline and significant mortality in older adults.[311]

Most primary psychiatric disorders and subclinical psychiatric conditions can affect memory and cognition. Depression, anxiety, and sleep disorders can cause lethargy and disorientation, memory loss, or other cognitive changes, and can also be a consequence of, or co-exist with, dementia.[65] Somatoform disorders (the group of psychiatric diagnoses characterized by physical symptoms that are not explained by biological factors, "sensitive self-monitoring," personality traits (like neuroticism), and even the fear of dementia can also prompt concerns about cognitive decline.

Neuropsychiatric symptoms (NPS) are present with all causes of dementia, and are described as "changes in personality, behavior, or comportment symptoms. These include uncharacteristic mood fluctuations such as agitation, loss of motivation, impaired initiative, apathy, loss of drive, social withdrawal, failing interest in previous activities, loss of empathy, compulsive or obsessive behaviors, and socially unacceptable behaviors. Conversion to dementia is significantly higher in patients with NPS."[362] With or without progression to dementia, NPS can lead to significant functional impairments.[98]

Mild behavioral impairment (MBI) is a specific late-life syndrome with prominent neuropsychiatric and behavioral symptoms, but without major cognitive changes.[363] The neuropsychiatric symptoms of MBI have been considered another marker of preclinical dementia, and occur with a frequency of around 10–15%, and more commonly in frontotemporal dementia (FTD).[98,363-365]

Diagnosing Uncommon Dementias

Beginning in medical school, providers are taught that the first step in uncovering any diagnosis is to "think of it," often by going down lists like those above to find a treatable or heritable form of dementia. With AD comprising more than three-quarters of dementia cases, the percentage of treatable or preventable needles in the dementia haystack is small.

However, the chance to mitigate the course of even a small percentage of so many elderly individuals would greatly benefit those patients and their families. As with Alzheimer's disease, very early ("pre-diagnostic") functional impairment and cognitive decline have also been recently noted in these less frequent neurodegenerative diseases. Identifying these before symptoms become obvious could improve selection for preventive and early disease-modifying treatment trials.[366] The standard medical history, family history, symptoms, and physical signs elicited in a comprehensive medical examination can narrow the list of possibilities.[124] Testing will vary with age and the clinician's degree of suspicion for non-AD causes like known metabolic disorders, HIV infection, cancer, autoimmune disease, or others.[65,124,366]

The bottom line: Acting oddly, forgetting, and progressive inability to care for oneself is not always Alzheimer's disease. Appropriate pursuit of alternative possibilities by a knowledgeable clinician can, in some cases, relieve suffering and restore some hope.

For an Overview of Alzheimer's Disease Treatments, See Chapter 5

Alzheimer's Disease: Progression and Prognosis[125]

Progression Is Variable and Unpredictable

Not everyone will progress from the asymptomatic, preclinical stage to SCD, then MCI, then AD. Those who develop dementia do not always experience the seven clinically recognizable stages described (in chapter 3) by Reisberg (from normal for age to vegetative).[177] Nor does everyone with AD experience outward expressions of the disease at the same rate or intensity as others.

Prognosis: Current AD treatments have not been found to increase survival or to definitively halt disease progression. Many patients die in the early or middle stages, while patients who live through the full course of the disease may survive for ten to twenty years. In a large Scandinavian study, the median survival time after a dementia diagnosis was 5.1 years for women and 4.3 years for men. Predictors of mortality were advanced age, male sex, comorbidity, worse cognitive function, a final diagnosis of non-Alzheimer dementia, living alone, and using more medications.[367]

End of Life Concerns: Advanced dementia is perceived as a terminal illness, with a similar symptom burden and prognosis to progressive cancer.[368] End-of-life considerations (life support, resuscitation, treatment of intercurrent illnesses, "comfort measures", etc.) should be discussed early in the course of AD to maximize understanding by all involved of the prognosis, plan, and available resources. The patient's priorities should be clearly documented and shared with family members, caretakers, and providers as well as formalized in medical advance directives and financial powers of attorney.[369]

How Do Dementia Patients Die?

AD is the fifth-leading cause of death among Americans age sixty-five and older.[227] Often, instead of listing AD on death certificates as a primary cause, the illness immediately preceding death, although technically a *complication* of Alzheimer's disease (and most commonly pneumonia), is often recorded instead. As a result, deaths from AD and related dementias are seriously underreported.

Also contributing to the inconsistency in identifying the cause of death in dementia sufferers is the frequent (and appropriate) decision against end-of-life medical intervention for conditions that may be potentially treatable in the short term, and for which intercession might temporarily delay death. It is often that unpredictable, and untreated "final straw" that is listed on a death certificate.

Causes of death uniquely associated with dementia include:

Suicide. A risk factor is the specific diagnosis of AD. Individuals identified as having dementia had a 54% higher risk of suicide within the first year after their diagnosis.[308] The risk of suicide was significantly increased in patients diagnosed with dementia before age sixty-five, in the first three months after diagnosis, and in patients with psychiatric comorbidities. Among those under age sixty-five and within three months of diagnosis, the suicide risk was nearly seven times higher than in patents without dementia.[370] Dementia also increased the risk of death by suicide within one year after diagnosis, compared to those without dementia, regardless of the presence of other mental disorders.[371]

Aspiration pneumonia. Because Alzheimer's causes healthy brain cells to die, vital connections are lost, including those to the muscles that control swallowing, continence, and mobility. As a result, those with Alzheimer's are at particular risk of choking or breathing food or liquid into their lungs (aspiration), which can cause difficult-to-treat pneumonias and death. Although tube feeding is often considered, no benefit has been found in persons with advanced dementia, and it is not recommended.[368,372,373]

Fatal complications from falls, immobility-related skin breakdown, and urinary infections are also common.

Coping with Alzheimer's

For Patients: Adjusting to Your Life with Memory Loss and Dementia[374]

Driving: Those with very mild AD may be able to drive, but a family member should ride along regularly to assure safety. Once the patient reaches the mild stage of AD (or when the family member is uncomfortable riding with the patient), driving should stop. If the patient does not want to stop driving, formal reevaluations for maintaining one's license to drive are available at most rehabilitation hospitals and Departments of Motor Vehicles. AARP offers significant information and resources on this topic.

Financial affairs: Patients with MCI and AD at any stage should have their financial affairs supervised and monitored by family members or legal representatives. These safeguards should include protection from telemarketers and other solicitations for money, and avoiding any independent investing.

Working is healthy from the patient's perspective but should be supervised. If problems in job performance were to occur, there should be no risks to the patient or others. Those with moderate to severe AD should not be left alone.

Layers of support: Home health aides and homemakers can help patients and benefit caregivers. Day programs offer a healthy routine and respite for the family. Call it a "club." Assisted living is ideal for patients who need more care than can be provided in a home without a caregiver present. Long-term care is necessary for almost all patients with dementia at some point in their illness. Units that specialize in dementia care are ideal. Families should be encouraged to plan ahead.

For Caregivers

Positive aspects of caregiving include developing a deeper appreciation for life, receiving satisfaction from living according to one's values and sense of duty, and a strengthening of their relationship with the person living with dementia. At the same time, caregivers face risks to their own physical and mental health, family conflict, social isolation, and negative consequences for their finances and livelihood.[375] *All caregivers benefit from general supportive measures*:

Listen: Caregivers are advised to find a network and other means for coping with challenges to their own physical and mental health. This can range from finding a primary care provider, to support groups, to babysitters.

Educate: Both caregivers and their patients benefit from a full understanding of the nature of the disease: stage, prognosis, treatments, trajectory, and sources that can provide answers.

Plan: You will need support for financial and legal issues and the next steps (adding and accepting help, transition to twenty-four-hour care.)[376]

Specific programs for at-home caregivers have included multiple behavioral interventions to improve caregiver well-being:[377]

- Counseling via telephone, online resources, or videos
- Mindfulness-based stress reduction techniques
- Care-management support systems utilizing clinical teams accessible via telephone or the internet.
- Standard evidence-based psychological therapies like anger and depression management, group

therapy, psychotherapy, education, multimodal (combined) approaches, and counseling for patient and the caregiver together.

Formal programs to support both caregivers and patients were analyzed by the Agency for Healthcare Research and Quality (AHRQ) in 2020[378] and the National Academies of Sciences, Engineering, and Medicine in 2021.[375]Two models were identified as somewhat helpful:

(1)   *Collaborative care models* employ multidisciplinary teams that integrate medical and psychosocial approaches to improve the quality of the patient's life, achieve guideline-based quality indicators, and reduce emergency room visits. Common components include coordinating psychosocial interventions, a care manager, care plans, case tracking, and collaboration with providers.

(2)   *REACH II* (Resources for Enhancing Alzheimer's Caregiver Health II), in various versions, is a multicomponent intervention to reduce caregiver burden. A combination of strategies includes education (problem-solving, skills training, stress management), personalized support (group discussions and role-playing in-home and phone-support sessions, and caregiver feedback). These programs may improve informal caregiver depression at six months.[377]

Maximizing family participation: "Family members are additional victims of all progressive dementias."[65] Approximately 70% of patients with Alzheimer's disease are cared for at home by a family member. The availability of family care varies with gender, race, and socioeconomic status. Adults with dementia and disability who have greater family availability were significantly more likely to receive informal care and less likely to use formal (paid) care.

The chance of a community-dwelling adult with dementia moving to a nursing home within two years was substantially lower for those who had a co-resident adult child (11%) compared with those who had at least one adult child living close by (20%), versus those whose children all lived far away (23%).[379]

Start discussions early. Begin simply by planning for aging in general: retirement, home remodeling for safety concerns and comfort, wills/estate planning, medical advance directives, assistive technology, downsizing, relocating, etc.

A recommendation from my personal life and my practice: For decades I have recommended *"The Complete Bedside Companion: A No-Nonsense Guide to Caring for the Seriously Ill"* by Robert J. McFarlane and Phillip Bashe.[380] I used to hand out copies of six typically enlightening pages from it to families of failing patients along with my recommendation that they consider buying the book. The content is exactly as described in the title.

The five-hundred-plus pages contain invaluable, practical advice, ranging from changing sheets on a bed with someone in it to "Preparing for the Worst." Energizing, organizing, and cooperating with family members is particularly well discussed. I have given away any number of copies, which today can readily be found, used, for two to five dollars online. If you are caring for anyone with a debilitating illness, I am comfortable that they will benefit from your reading and sharing this book. Two more recent references specific to Alzheimer's disease are recommended by the authors of the very latest AD textbook. It may be worth a look.[43,381,382]

The realities of current caregiving options should be at the forefront of discussions.[117] The caregiver shortage affects every alternative. Given a choice, most of us would likely prefer being cared for at home for as long as possible. Family is often seen as ideal, but practical and financial considerations are limiting for many. Frank discussions about family-member capabilities and limitations, including financial, should occur early.

Medicaid pays for most long-term care services in the United States. If elders are not currently on Medicaid, and the situation is such that Medicaid-funded long-term care is a primary consideration, get expert advice early. Ease into information sharing with the patient and among family members.

Sharing responsibilities: Start going along to doctor's appointments and distributing duties around finances, such as banking, bill paying, and investing. Build a safety net to protect all involved against fraud, accidents, or memory failure, particularly co-signatures, securing credit/debit cards, trusts, and powers of attorney. Consider electronic or mechanical resources: pill boxes, audio or video monitoring, voice assistants, panic buttons, and motion sensors.

Caring: Don't underestimate the value to the patient of the little things that anyone can do. Suggest activities that do not require preplanning or ongoing commitments of time or money. In addition, even a brief respite provided to caregivers by others can facilitate a valuable reset and recharge. These sorts of activities are perfect when a friend or neighbor calls, writes, or stops by and asks, "What can I do to help?"

When asked "What can I do?" here are some good answers:

- "Visit": in person, via video, FaceTime or phone call. Reminisce, recall "blasts from the past" (be creative, you know the person best).

- Sit and listen or read the paper, a magazine, or a book together.
- Make contact: Hold hands. Hug. Get the patient out of bed to a chair, maybe to another room, a different window, another view.
- Get moving: Take a walk or ride. Make a meal together. Dress up.
- Simulate or find comforting favorites (foods, music, photo albums, home videos, movies, games, memorabilia).
- Pet visits.

Exploring the Full Spectrum of Care—From Home to Hospice[383,384]

Give early thought to maximizing caregiving at home, which provides optimal initial support to the patient and family. Assistance may include home health aides,[385] Meals on Wheels, or a visiting nurse. Consider structured activities outside of the home, such as adult day care ("respite care") and social or exercise programs.

The best care I have personally witnessed and would want for myself is from carefully selected personnel supported, managed, and supervised by a home-care professional and an involved family. This can add years of improved quality of life but is not currently an option for those with even moderate means.

Progress in supporting home care is being made. Some states have enacted expanded paid family leave laws. Others have compensation mechanisms for caregivers and caregiver training *(AARP Bulletin, November 2023)*. There are calls to Congress to change the proportions of Medicaid and Medicare spending to allow seniors to age safely at home. Support these efforts!

At some point, escalating physical needs, symptom burden, and behavioral disturbances will challenge the continuation of in-home care. Use the time acquired from maximizing home-based care in the early stages of the disease to anticipate future requirements. This includes considering full-time in-home arrangements and outside-the-home options (assisted living or a skilled nursing facility).[65]

Long-term Care: Nursing homes can be less than eager to accept those living with AD. These patients often require longer stays, have a lower likelihood of discharge, require more staff time because of their clinical and behavioral complexities, and use fewer therapy hours, generating less revenue per bed.[384]

Hospice and palliative care, a primary source of end-of-life comfort for Medicare beneficiaries, is less often available to dementia patients because of the uncertain timeframe of their prognosis. For those with medical diseases, hospice eligibility requires less than six months' life expectancy. Specific helpful references include "Expert Advice for Finding the Right Home Health Aide"[385] and "Understanding Nursing Home, Hospice, and Palliative Care for Individuals with Later-Stage Dementia."[384]

Legal Issues in Memory Loss and Dementia[386]

"Capacity" is the ability to understand and make the decisions and judgments necessary to sign legal documents. Capacity depends on (1) the nature of the deliberation needed to fully understand the ramifications of consenting and signing, (2) the degree of impairment, and (3) the level of agreement among the family.

In medical settings, the focus is most often on a patient's "decision-making capacity," the ability to give informed consent or refusal to medical interventions or surgical procedures.[387]

Important legal issues include wills, trusts, general powers of attorney for financial affairs, guardianship, and a living will (a.k.a., "Advance Directive" or "Power of Attorney for Healthcare").

To be clear, there is no legal advice intended or offered here.
Individual circumstances will vary widely.
Ultimately, seek professional guidance.

Chapter 5
CURRENT TREATMENTS FOR ALZHEIMER'S DISEASE

AD Treatment:
Wait for it! . . . .
No, literally, wait for it.

Treatment Overview: Alzheimer's Disease

The Harsh Realities

The goal for research into any illness is an "effective, approved, disease-modifying treatment."

AD remains the only major cause of mortality without one.

"Disease-modifying" means "potentially curative;" i.e., able to reverse the course of Alzheimer's disease. Current therapies, if effective, only "slow progression." "The development of effective drugs is a difficult and time-consuming process, accompanied by a very high failure rate."[192,390,391] As evidence of those longstanding challenges, there were no new drugs approved for AD between 2003 and 2021.[392]

The U. S. Preventive Services Task Force (USPSTF) is an independent volunteer panel of national experts in disease prevention and evidence-based medicine. Their mandate is to "improve the health of people nationwide by making evidence-based recommendations about clinical preventive services." Their 2020 review of treatments for AD included an examination of over twenty thousand scientific publications. Among their conclusions were: "The benefits [of Alzheimer's treatment] are quite small and likely not of clinical significance."[388,389] Unlike many other organs in the body, brain cells do not regenerate. Once a brain cell is lost, it is gone forever. As more brain cells die, the disease progresses and more abilities are lost.

With respect to specific treatments, the USPSTF summarized their findings as follows:

> In general, there is support that AChEIs [the 3 approved cholinesterase inhibitors, donepezil (Aricept®), rivastigmine (Exelon®), and galantamine (Razadyne®)] plus memantine (Namenda®)) and interventions that support caregivers, including those that help coordinate care for patients and caregivers, *can result in small improvements in the short term.*
>
> Unfortunately, *the average effects of these benefits are quite small and likely not of clinical significance.* [emphasis added]. Any benefits are further limited by the commonly experienced side effects of medications and the limited availability of complex caregiver interventions. Cognitive stimulation and training, exercise interventions, and other medications and supplements showed some favorable effects on patients' cognitive and physical function, but trial evidence lacked consistency and the estimates of benefit were imprecise."[389]

Alzheimer's disease treatments are most often spoken of by clinicians as "experimental" or "encouraging" or "coming soon." Even the latest (2022) textbook on AD, when considering "Why Diagnose and Treat Dementia?" identifies the effect of existing treatments solely as "turning back the clock on *memory* loss" and *does not mention cognitive loss!* Symptom control certainly helps patients and caregivers. Delaying progression may save money, and an accurate diagnosis defines prognosis and improves planning. Regarding treatment and cure since 2003: "New, disease-modifying treatments are being developed and may be available soon."[43]

Since it became clear that the underlying pathophysiological processes of AD begin many years before the onset of dementia, the hope was that identifying patients in the preclinical stages of AD would lead to interventions that could delay or perhaps even prevent the emergence of the clinical syndrome. Repeated failures to develop disease-modifying treatments for identified Alzheimer's patients have led to suggestions that disease-specific therapies be directed at much earlier stages of AD, before symptoms, and perhaps even for *prevention* in those at high risk. A persistent question has been: "So why do we keep testing drugs aimed at the initial stages of the disease process in patients at the end-stage of the illness?"[393]

The very latest treatments, those unveiled since 2021 and followed through the summer of 2023, are anti-amyloid antibodies, discussed later in this chapter.

Clinical Trials of New (Experimental) Drugs

Although currently approved medications do not alter the disease process, they may have value in improving symptoms. Even successful experimental trials offering the first new options in decades provide (per the USPSTF above) only "small improvements in the short term."[389]

Are Clinical Trials for You?

Even though clinical trials are frequently mentioned by providers when discussing AD treatment options, drug experiments have so far offered little long-term benefit to patients. An example of the vague arguments made by researchers in favor of clinical trial participation is a 2022 National Public Radio (NPR) interview with Dr. Pierre Tariot, director of the Banner Alzheimer's Institute in Phoenix, Arizona.

Dr. Tariot optimistically refers to "a growing number of treatment options," but only mentioned two: (1) Aduhelm®, the highly controversial Alzheimer's drug approved in 2021 by the US Food and Drug Administration, but denied approval in Europe (see "Pharmacologic treatments" on page 160) and was later withdrawn in the US, and (2) the availability of a "range of clinical trials of experimental Alzheimer's drugs."[394] In reassuring the NPR audience that experimental treatments are the future of medicine (and the pharmaceutical industry, although not necessarily in that order), he fails to mention the fact that what is being tested are compounds that have not been approved by the FDA for your doctor to use or your pharmacist to sell. Also note that, in clinical trials, subjects may have up to a 50–50 chance of getting a sugar pill (placebo).

My opinion: Fingers crossed! Be sure to take those experimental pills (or placebos) with a hefty measure of salt. I have valued, studied, critically reviewed, conducted, and participated in human and animal research for over fifty-five years. Such efforts remain the only hope of progress to improve understanding, find new treatments, or discover a cure. I encourage readers to strongly consider clinical trial participation and will consider doing so again myself.

However, I am compelled to provide an alternative perspective to that offered by those whose goal is to recruit
you. Let mine be the most objective voice in the room
with you, your family, and the white-coated authority figures offering hope (along with lengthy and incomprehen-
sible consent forms to sign). In my opinion, one's choice
to participate in an Alzheimer's disease experimental drug
trial should be viewed more as a gift with potential value
to future generations, rather than a likely benefit for oneself. When the success rate of proposed AD treatments
over the last two decades has been so dismal that the only
choices presented are between unproven options and
placebos, do your best to calculate the benefit <u>to you!</u>

<u>Which will you prefer: the cup half full, or the one</u>
<u>half empty?</u>

Generally Achievable Goals of Currently Available AD Interventions[43]

There is evidence that *risk factor modification* is worthwhile. A
healthy lifestyle is most often suggested, and is always a good
idea.[115] In recent years, the incidence of dementia has declined
in Europe and North America, supporting the view that
dementia risk in late life is modifiable. Evidence suggests that
intervention strategies that promote general health, maintain
vascular health, and increase cognitive reserve are likely to help
preserve cognitive function till late in life, approaching the goal
of aging without dementia![334]

There are also shorter-term treatment benefits. While memory loss cannot be halted or reversed to where it was before AD,
current treatments can "turn the clock back" for some to where

they were six to twelve months previously. So far, nothing can stop the clock from ticking down, nor slow its rate.[395] Available treatments can address and improve *symptoms* of Alzheimer's disease and associated conditions (anxiety, depression, agitation, aggression). In patients with advanced dementia, providing comfort only can still be a worthwhile primary goal.

Currently Available Drugs for Alzheimer's Disease

It is important to distinguish between Alzheimer's disease treatments and the much larger body of remedies marketed to relieve or delay the consequences of natural aging (senior moments, age-related cognitive decline (ARCD), etc.), that are *not* early AD.[183] Presently, "The purpose of Alzheimer's medication is to slow progression of the disease, as there is currently no cure."[147] As of mid-2023, there were seven FDA-approved prescription medications for AD that operate via three mechanisms of action. See https://www.alz.org /alzheimers-dementia/treatments/medications-for-memory#how.

The Latest Treatments: Anti-Amyloid Monoclonal Antibodies

The "amyloid cascade" is a widely accepted hypothesis proposing that the neurodegeneration and resultant dementia of AD occur as a result of the formation and accumulation of toxic beta-amyloid proteins in our brains.[396] Monoclonal antibodies against amyloid are currently among the most actively investigated, potentially disease-modifying therapies targeting the biology of Alzheimer's disease. Since 2005, more than one hundred trials have been registered to study the effect of monoclonal antibodies in patients with MCI or AD.[397]

Aducanumab (Aduhelm®), the first available anti-amyloid agent, has been controversial since the hearings for FDA approval in 2021. A monoclonal antibody given by intravenous infusion, Aduhelm® directly targets beta amyloid,[398] and was initially priced at $56,000 per patient.[399] Criticisms of the drug's release included[400,401]:

(1) Efficacy trials were stopped early because of futility.
(2) Based on only a single trial, aducanumab was approved by the FDA despite *a 10:0 vote against* such approval by their own scientific advisory panel. Three panel members resigned after the FDA authorized it anyway, and a subsequent congressional investigation raised "serious concerns" about the FDA's process in this case.
(3) Serious side effects (brain swelling and brain hemorrhage) and the additional cost and risks associated with those complications, occurred in over one-third of patients receiving the drug.[402]
(4) The enormous cost burden on families and on Medicare, especially since "there is no prospect of curing Alzheimer's disease or restoring cognitive function with aducanumab."[401] The US Centers for Medicare and Medicaid Services declined to cover aducanumab under federal insurance plans unless a person is enrolled in a clinical trial.
(5) *Aduhelm®* was denied approval by the European Medicines Agency (the European Union's equivalent of the US FDA).

Criticisms of the FDA's process were:

(1) Too fast.
(2) Ignoring the advisory panel lowers the standards of scientific evidence used for drug approvals, and requires clinicians to scrutinize approved medications much more carefully.[401,403]

(3)   The cost of aducanumab is a "shocking discrimination against everyone with Alzheimer's disease, especially those who are already disproportionately impacted by this fatal disease, including women, Blacks and Hispanics." (from The Alzheimer's Association)[404]

(4)   Ethical challenges for neurologists, patients and families: There is incomplete data available to guide aducanumab prescribing. Concerns include "the prospect of worrisome conflicts of interest, and the financial and practical burdens that using aducanumab will impose. (from[401] and the American Academy of Neurology)" Patients and families will want it, and some otherwise skeptical physicians will feel bound to educate, and then honor those wishes in order to "preserve patient autonomy."[405]

(5)   Aducanumab availability could hinder enrollment in clinical trials of more effective interventions.

UPDATE: Aducanumab was withdrawn from the US market by the manufacturer in January 2024.

I wouldn't take it if they gave me the $56,000.

Lecanemab (Leqembi™): In late 2022, Lecanemab became the second, and so far, more positively received, available anti-amyloid agent. It received FDA approval for the treatment of patients with mild cognitive impairment (MCI) or the mild dementia stage of Alzheimer's disease with confirmed beta-amyloid. Subsequently, CMS determined that Medicare would largely assume payment for eligible seniors. Leqembi™ was described by some as the product of "the first successful, completed, Phase 3 Alzheimer's drug study in the Western world in more than 20 years," finding *"modestly less decline"* [emphasis added] in cognition and function in the Lecanemab group than with a placebo over eighteen months, in the Lecanemab group, along with "very real side effects" similar to Aducanumab, including brain swelling and bleeding.[406]

The degree of enthusiasm with which such preliminary findings have been welcomed is a measure of how desperate patients, families, doctors, and drug companies have been for a potentially disease-modifying breakthrough in Alzheimer's treatment.

The most comprehensive meta-analysis available by May 2023 evaluated the efficacy of Lecanemab compared with a placebo in patients with mild or early AD concluded that, "Further studies are needed . . .with a large sample size and an extended period to evaluate whether Lecanemab could be utilized as a potential disease-modifying treatment for advanced AD patients."[407] Cost at the time of initial release was $26,500/year.

Unlike with aducanumab, there were few questions about the quality of the underlying Lecanemab research. Concerns centered around whether the size of the *statistically* significant effects on cognitive decline measured over large *groups* of patients would translate into "clinically meaningful" benefits for *individual* patients over time.[408-410]

The initial answer, in a subsequent review and meta-analysis of Lecanemab's safety and efficacy in four randomized controlled trials involving 3,108 AD patients concluded that "actual clinical significance is still to be established."[407]

Donanemab is the latest in this group of anti-amyloid agents. As of March, 2024, with application for FDA approval still pending, results of the donanemab Phase 3 clinical trial in more than 1,700 persons and initially reported in an Eli Lilly press release,[411] have been peer-reviewed and published.[412]

A reminder: the FDA assesses three phases of clinical research before approval of new drugs. Phase 1: Safety and dosage studies in <100 people with or without the condition; Phase 2: up to several hundred people with the disease looking at efficacy and side effects; and Phase 3: 300–3,000 people with the disease studied over one to four years years for efficacy and monitoring of adverse reactions.

Results: Forty-seven percent of participants on donanemab showed no decline at one year on summed Clinical Dementia Rating Scales (CDR-SB), a measure of disease severity, compared to 29% of participants on placebo, p<0. 001. Clearance of amyloid plaque (a criterion for stopping the monthly antibody infusions) occurred in 52% of participants by one year and in 72% by eighteen months. Participants on donanemab had 40% less decline in ability to perform activities of daily living at eighteen months, and a 39% lower risk of progressing to the next stage of disease compared to placebo.[411-413]

Critiques focus largely on the difficulty of assuring true *clinical* significance from the small, but statistically significant differences observed between those receiving donanemab and the placebo group. The greater the numbers of subjects in study groups, the more common it is for small numeric differences in group averages to achieve "statistical significance." *Statistical* significance commonly means that observed differences between experimental and control or placebo groups had less than a 5% probability of occurring by chance. It is usually up to expert opinion and different sorts of experiments to ascertain whether small differences achieve *clinical* significance (i.e., there is *real value to patients* in that small numeric change).

For example, the absolute difference between treatment and placebo groups on one measure (the "CDR-SB scale") was just under 0.7. Some researchers argue it takes at least a full point on that scale to represent a clear difference in disease severity.[411] Similarly, changes over time in the composite score on the Integrated Alzheimer's Disease Rating Scale (which ranges from 0 to 144) identified a statistically significant between-group difference of just 3.2 points (2%) in favor of donanemab, a difference that was questionably relevant clinically.[414] In an analysis of Phase 2 data, Wessels et al. (2023) determined that treatment with donanemab would delay "clinically meaningful worsening" in cognitive and functional abilities of Alzheimer's patients by approximately six months."[415]

Does 6–12 Months Remain the Limit of AD Therapeutic Benefit in 2023?

The six-month delay in clinical worsening attributable to donanemab echoes the very first page of Budson and Solomon's 2022, 276-page 2nd edition of **Memory Loss, Alzheimer's Disease and Dementia**.[43] Writing more generally about their experience with the drugs in use for the last several decades, and preceding the donanemab studies, they said: "Current pharmacologic treatments for Alzheimer's disease have been shown to be able to "turn the clock back" on memory loss for 6 to 12 months."[395] In general, regardless of the drug used, positive treatment effects on memory are more often reported than benefits to cognition or dementia.

The major *complications* of anti-amyloid therapy are "Amyloid-Related Imaging Abnormalities (ARIA)" seen on MRI. Not always symptomatic and found to a lesser degree in untreated AD, they are most commonly observed as temporary swelling in an area or areas of the brain (ARIA-E) or as micro-hemorrhages or superficial blood staining (ARIA-H). "Serious" ARIA occurred in 1.6% of donanemab-treated patients with three deaths.[413] In their systematic review and meta-analysis addressing the safety and efficacy of monoclonal antibodies for Alzheimer's disease, Lacorte et al., showed an overall higher risk of both ARIA-E and ARIA-H in patients treated with antibodies compared to placebo.[397] They noted the absence of data on the potential long-term consequences of these antibody-related increases in brain swelling and hemorrhage. A prior longitudinal study on families with dominantly inherited AD did report that the presence of cerebral microhemorrhages predicted a faster decline of dementia rating scores.[416] The potential effect of ARIA on the natural history of the disease remains unclear.

The early bottom line on AD treatments with anti-amyloid monoclonal antibodies:

(1) Anti-amyloid monoclonal antibodies *do* significantly reduce the brain's amyloid burden.[397] However, the role of amyloid load as a surrogate marker for cognitive decline has been called into question.[417] After analyzing pooled results from fourteen randomized controlled trials of anti-amyloid drugs for prevention or treatment of AD, Ackley, et al.(2021) concluded that *"amyloid reduction strategies do not substantially improve cognition."*[418] "Currently available evidence does not support a clear link between amyloid load and cognitive performance, suggesting that reducing the amyloid

load might have low-to-no effect in improving cognitive performance or slowing cognitive decline."[397]

(2) The effect of current anti-amyloid monoclonal antibodies on Alzheimer's disease, if any, is limited to slowing progression slightly, and perhaps "turning back the clock" of memory loss for six months. "To date [August 2021], four monoclonal antibodies that target Aβ (beta-amyloid) have been shown to have no benefit on cognition in their original phase 2/3 clinical trials in Alzheimer's disease."[419]

(3) Unlike when we attempt to treat other deadly diseases, "in dementia treatment, survival has never been measured as a benefit. Instead, we speak of living longer in a certain state of mind. The measures we use—cognition and day-to-day function—and the significance of changes in them aren't readily understandable."[420]

(4) There are reproducible risks of brain swelling and hemorrhage with as-yet unknown long-term consequences.

(5) There is a significant lack of agreement on effectiveness. As of May 2023, responses to studies of anti-amyloid antibodies published in peer-reviewed medical journals range from "Transformative Treatments that Redefine Alzheimer's Disease"[421] to "Still grasping at straws. . . clinical trials with these agents should be abandoned."[422] In the middle of the range is *Science* (May 14, 2023): "Latest Alzheimer's antibody is 'not a miracle drug.' Results on Eli Lilly's donanemab highlight stark risk-benefit trade-offs."[411] No anti-amyloid drug reverses

or repairs brain damage already caused by the disease, so many Alzheimer's experts consider them to be only a first step in a potentially fruitful direction.[403] "Whether the harms of these drugs are balanced by their modest clinical benefits will ultimately require more data."[423]

(6) In 2024 we are still largely dealing with press releases and preliminary results from the developers of the drugs. Press releases are particularly prone to excited but unsupported optimism. Confirmatory studies and longer-term outcomes will be coming.

Just reflect on the "good news/bad news" cycling of opinion and publicity regarding the hazards versus benefits of common temptations like red meat, wine, coffee, eggs, alcohol, chocolate, and others. New revelations and reversals identified by another long-term study come every few years. To quote myself from elsewhere in the book: "Remember when 'good cholesterol' was an oxymoron?"

---

(7) Recent declines in AD in developed countries are not explained by any decrease in the number of amyloid plaques present at the end of life. The fact that brain amyloid concentrations remain stable in spite of trends towards less end-of-life dementia raises questions regarding the value of the new anti-amyloid drugs.[424]

(8) One highly respected director of an Alzheimer's center in a major university described the FDA's preliminary approval of lecanemab in this way:

"Over the past several months, my conversations with colleagues in the Alzheimer's field have featured an unusual sentiment: optimism infected with worry. *Optimism* because, after years of failed studies and the disastrous accelerated approval of aducanumab, we're enjoying a less than one-year-old streak of good news." *The worry*: "Lecanemab and donanemab present the same risks to the brain: microscopic hemorrhages and swelling. At the FDA advisory committee meeting, the discussion of these side effects' likelihood and how best to mitigate them was thoughtful but incomplete."[420]

I have never treated Alzheimer's disease. Having loved persons with dementia, and fearing it myself, I would give anything to be more positive about the latest "break-throughs." Scientists and clinicians will often differ in their assessments, and studies will vary in their rigor. With such a huge and growing body of information, no one can analyze it all. My interpretation is based on the more than five hundred published scientific reports that I have read and cited here. Fifty-seven percent of those references are from 2020 or later.

New Treatments = (same side effects) + (very high cost) + (unknown long-term benefit) + (zero patient improvement and only "modestly less decline")

Yet the combination of an eighteen-year drought in new Alzheimer's drug approvals, coupled with decades of failed trials, seems to have left the widely diverse "Alzheimer's Community" (doctors, patients, families, researchers, funders, medical centers, drug companies, nursing homes, jellyfish farmers, the "memory care" industry, insurance companies, and more) ever more desperate for any positive news. Despite so many disappointing AD "advances," hope springs eternal. A kind of desperate enthusiasm seems to amplify any positive spin, overpowering more temperate appraisals.

If I'm going to bet (what's left of) my brain on a new drug . . . I'm going to need some convincing beyond my latest eminent neurologist's January 2023 (accurate) description of the donanemab Phase 3 press release as showing a "relatively modest slowing down of the course (of AD)" and "1–2% risk" (of presumably serious ARIA). There are literally thousands of brilliant people working on this and other approaches. As yet, my opinion remains: "Let's wait a little longer and see."

Current "Standard" Therapies in Use for Decades

The benefits and limitations of the following are well known:

Cholinesterase inhibitors:[425] Alzheimer's disease is linked to a deficiency of brain acetylcholine (Ach), a "neurotransmitter" that carries signals from one brain cell to another. The cholinesterase inhibitors prevent the natural breakdown of acetylcholine, increasing its concentrations in the areas of the brain important for memory and other cognitive functions. Three of the four medications previously approved by the FDA for treatment of AD—donepezil (Aricept), rivastigmine (Exelon) and galantamine (Razadyne)—employ this mechanism of action. And yes, they all do slow down the clinical progression of mild-to-moderate AD by improving the symptoms. However, they do *not* affect the accumulation of destructive brain proteins.

It is helpful that these inhibitors can stabilize cognition, modify behavior and improve global function and participation in activities of daily living (ADLs). Improved symptoms can delay nursing home placement, and reduce both health care expenditures and caregiver burdens for patients with AD. However, the effects are modest, and they are not apparent in some individuals.[65]

Glutamate regulator: Memantine (Namenda®)[426] also affects brain chemical messengers (neurotransmitters). It enhances release of glutamate and stimulates dopamine transmission, both of which are considered critical for learning and memory. Prescribed to improve memory, attention, reason, language, and the ability to perform simple tasks, Memantine was approved by the FDA in 2003 for treatment of moderate-to-severe Alzheimer's disease.

The combination of the two types, a cholinesterase inhibitor and a glutamate regulator (Namzaric®: donepezil plus memantine) is believed to have greater effectiveness in slowing the progression of AD, and is approved for moderate-to-severe Alzheimer's disease. The most recent AD text concludes that Namzaric® improves attention, alertness, apathy, and global functioning (but not memory per se), and that a combination therapy gives the best short- and long-term outcomes in patients with moderate to severe Alzheimer's dementia.[426] Common side effects include dizziness, agitation, headache, and confusion.

What about MCI? Neither cholinesterase inhibitors nor memantine are indicated for mild cognitive impairment. These drugs do not alter the progression of MCI to dementia.[125]

The Alzheimer's Drug Development "Pipeline"

Development of new therapies for diseases of the nervous system has historically been challenging, with high failure rates and long development times. So much so that some major pharmaceutical companies stopped investing in this area of drug development. All current clinical trials in the United States are registered with https://clinicaltrials.gov. "As of January 25, 2022 there were 143 agents in 172 clinical trials for AD. Of the 3-phases of drug development and testing, only 31 were in Phase 3." Disease-modifying therapies were 83% of the total number of agents in trials; symptomatic cognitive-enhancing treatments represent 10%, while drugs intended for the treatment of neuropsychiatric symptoms comprised 7%.[392]

Non-Pharmacologic (Behavioral) Strategies for Treatment of Alzheimer's Disease

Non-drug interventions focus on symptom control through behavior modification, and on maintaining physical strength via nutrition and physical therapy, rather than on memory or cognition.[147] Behavioral and "non-pharmacologic approaches for treating the symptoms of AD can improve function as well as or better than medication."[427]

Behavioral treatments can help compensate for memory loss, and are recommended before moving to potent drugs such as antidepressants, antipsychotics, and sedatives to control agitation and other behavioral symptoms.[428] Recent trials of antidepressants and atypical antipsychotics for agitation and other behavioral symptoms in Alzheimer's disease showed no benefit over placebo or "treatment as usual."[429,430] Although supported only by "encouraging but inconclusive" evidence, increased physical activity, valuable to the elderly in so many ways, is seemingly beneficial in delaying or slowing age-related cognitive decline (ARCD), not dementia.[183]

"Health systems would be well advised to focus on providing good-quality, nondrug psychosocial care and support for those with agitation in dementia rather than seeking to use medication to deal with these complex states."[429] Psychiatric symptoms and behavioral problems in those patients who are easily distressed or psychotic may respond to "The 3 R's":[65,428]

(1) Reassure: When the limitation of an important activity may be involved, the caregiver should be ready to reassure the patient that there will be a variety of ways in which the patient can continue doing what they like to do.

(2) Reconsider: Put yourself in the position of the patient: If it were you, would things look positive?, negative? restrictive? permissive?

(3) Redirect: Try to shift the patient to another activity that he or she can accomplish independently and that will distract them.

External memory aids and environmental cues such as calendars, a (big) clock, lists, and whiteboards providing reorientation to the environment can be very reassuring and help keep patients functional. It is important to keep such memory aids in the same place. Clear communication should be emphasized. Content should be simple and to the point. Given how common diminished hearing is in the elderly, speaking clearly and loudly is essential.

Learning new habits using *procedural memory* (as in learning to ride a bicycle, see chapter 1) allows patients with even moderate Alzheimer's disease to improve their function. Pictures are remembered better than words. Music can be helpful at all stages. Social and cognitively stimulating activities, as found in an enriched environment, have been shown to improve function.

Perhaps the most unique example of "enriched environments" is found in so-called "dementia villages." Much more prevalent worldwide than in the US, these facilities (both residential and nonresidential) design streets and even entire villages with a 1950s look. Directed at baby boomers, it is thought that such environments help dementia patients revisit happier times from their past. Some offer options among multiple "lifestyles" for seniors to choose the kind of food, art, music and furniture they were once accustomed to.[431]

For those to whom this may appeal, it could partially be done at home: a "nostalgia" bedroom and/or sitting room with furniture, wall art, photos, music, recorded or streamed older TV shows and the like. Check garage sales, thrift stores, and those dusty boxes in family attics for props and memorabilia.

Drug Treatments for Behavioral and Psychological Symptoms of Dementia

Behavioral symptoms of AD include apathy, depression, irritability, anxiety, aggression, agitation, psychosis, sleep disturbance and disinhibition or perseveration. Given the inability to cure AD, successfully modulating these symptoms will benefit patients, families, and caregivers. If possible, try non-pharmacological and behavioral interventions (page 172) before considering potent drugs like antidepressants, antipsychotics, and sedatives. These may result in significant drug vs. drug interactions and undesirable side effects. Before initiating medication for behavioral and psychological symptoms, be sure that the symptoms are not from medical conditions like a urinary infection or pneumonia, or being triggered by environmental circumstances.[65,428,432]

The use of psychiatric medications in the elderly with dementia can be controversial and requires a complete risk/benefit analysis. Medications (generally classified as "atypical antipsychotics") that are currently available to address such symptoms in Alzheimer's patients are potent, with significant associated side effects and adverse reactions. They are *specifically not approved by the FDA for use in elderly patients with dementia* because of reports of small but statistically significant increased risks of stroke and death when used in that population.

Such "off-label" use may be considered after a thorough discussion of the risks and potential benefits with patients and their families. When implemented judiciously by physicians skilled in treating Alzheimer's disease, irritability and depressive symptoms have been treated effectively with antidepressants, with the choice of agent based principally on side effects. Caregivers need to read and keep that densely printed brochure that comes from the pharmacy with the drug, be vigilant, and discuss any questions or possible adverse reactions with the pharmacist and your doctor.

"In general, such agents should be used only when necessary. Psychosis does not require treatment unless it leads to dangerous behavior, causes distress to the patient, or is disruptive to the family or other caregivers. When such agents are used, choosing lower doses and titrating upward slowly is advised. Once target symptoms are controlled, it is prudent to consider tapering off the medications after 2–3 months to determine whether longer-term treatment is necessary. Indeed, with longer-term treatment, benefits are less clear-cut and risks of severe adverse outcomes increase."[65]

Be grateful for any improvements in symptoms with these medications, but don't confuse a response of symptoms to therapy with successful treatment of the underlying disease. In general, such agents should be used only when necessary for the *patient's* benefit. Don't over-drug these folks (or allow others to do so) to make you feel better, or to keep them quiet and controlled for caregivers or nursing home staff. Sedation has its own serious side effects, like aspiration, depression, falls, bedsores, and worsening of cognition, awareness, and associated quality of life.

Preventing Cognitive Decline and Dementia: The Evidence Is "Encouraging but Inconclusive"

This is the judgement of the two most recent and comprehensive government-sponsored reviews of decades of research (and totaling nearly nine hundred pages).[182,183] Regarding prevention, the authors offer "some degree of support for the benefit of three classes of intervention: cognitive training, blood pressure management in people with hypertension, and increased physical activity."[183]

"Cognitive training" is used to describe a broad set of interventions to assist problem solving, memory, speed of processing and in identifying visual information on a screen. The largest such training effort to prevent cognitive decline and dementia was the ten-year ACTIVE trial, studying 2,800 "diverse . . . independent and vital elderly" participants, with an average age of seventy-four years.[433,434] Subjects were either assigned to a "no-contact control group" or specifically trained over five to six weeks (plus two subsequent "booster" sessions) on cognitive tasks requiring memory, reasoning, or speedy information processing, like learning a language and increasing proficiency in daily activities, such as playing bridge and doing crossword puzzles.[182,183]

When studied five years later, cognitive training showed no effect on the rate of new diagnoses of dementia in their study population.[433] *Ten years later*, when compared to control group participants, the majority of individuals who received cognitive training were functioning at or above their baseline level *for the trained ability*. The effects of training had persisted for a decade, but maintenance or improvement was only seen in the *specific tasks* on which they had been previously trained and tested. On those particular skills, 60%–70% of participants were as well or better off than when they started, and at least 60% reported less difficulty performing ADLs compared to 49% of non-trained participants.[434] Attempts to transfer any benefits of cognitive

176

training from one task to another have had poor success. *Only direct practice on the same specific test was able to improve scores on that test.*[435] When computers deliver "brain-training," there is no evidence to support any beneficial long-term cognitive effects.[183]

Efforts to develop, research, promote, (and sell) techniques or devices to ward off "cognitive decline" continue in our setting of enormous demand. In evaluating any new approaches, it is important to differentiate between those claiming to improve cognition in those with Alzheimer's disease from interventions targeting age-related cognitive decline (ARCD, a.k.a. "normal cognitive aging"). As an example, while increased physical activity may benefit ARCD, it has not been shown to have a significant impact on preventing dementia.[436]

Other recommended general treatments and lifestyle interventions have included removing potentially harmful medications, managing blood pressure, limiting alcohol intake, and diagnosing and treating any underlying sleep disorder.[65,183,320]

Vitamins, Minerals, Antioxidants, Anti-Inflammatories, Herbs, and Supplements[437]

Certain dietary substances have some scientific evidence in their favor and no clear harm attached to their use. There are ways to integrate supplements, alternative diets, and over-the-counter agents safely and intelligently into your overall health and fitness regime. A primary risk is in taking these *instead of* medical evaluation for problems of memory or cognition or taking them and excluding the health-care provider's recommended therapies.

Multivitamins: In recently published large-scale, long-term, randomized controlled trials daily multivitamin use (specifically Centrum Silver) was a "safe and readily available intervention" to protect cognitive function (i.e., ARCD) [438] and memory[439] in older adults.

As I have written in more than one section of this book, including "How to Play it Safe in the Supplement Aisle" (page 186), if your choice (of supplement) is based on published research, be sure of three things: (1) The research is published in a legitimate journal, (2) the recommended agent is essentially harmless, and (3) its alleged beneficial effects appear to be supported. The study mentioned above checks all those boxes for me, and I have changed my multivitamin of choice accordingly.

Carotenoids are a class of dietary antioxidants found in the yellow, orange, and red pigments produced by some plants, algae, and fungi. The body converts them into vitamins. In a study of more than seven thousand participants aged forty-five to ninety, serum levels of two specific carotenoids obtained at the beginning of the study, were associated with reduced risk of all-cause dementia over an average of sixteen years of observation.[440]

Curcumin is a component of turmeric, a relative of ginger, which is a golden-orange spice used for hundreds of years to add color, flavor, and nutrition to foods. Also utilized in various forms of traditional medicine in China and India, curcumin is believed to have multiple bio-pharmacological properties including strong antioxidant and anti-inflammatory effects. Currently under study for potential benefit in neurodegenerative diseases, animal studies and *in vitro* experiments have been promising. Human studies are limited and inconsistent. Bioavailability is a concern, as specific plant sources of curcumin vary considerably in content and absorption.[441-443]

Flavonoids are antioxidants found in strawberries, oranges, grapefruits, citrus juices, apples, pears, celery, peppers, and bananas. Increased intake of these dietary flavonols (1) has led to improved cognitive performance in both healthy young adults[444] and healthy older adults;[445-447] (2) was significantly associated with lower odds of SCD and better later-life subjective cognitive function;[59,60] and (3) may affect risk of ADRD (Alzheimer's disease and related dementias) in middle-aged and older adults by reducing a biomarker strongly associated with ADRD.[448]

> My favorite military communications acronym, which is acceptable in mixed company, is BLUF. That stands for "Bottom Line Up Front." Therefore, I concur with my mother (who passed away at ninety-eight with her faculties intact), and with the millions of parents before and after her: "Everything is good in moderation."

To Be Avoided

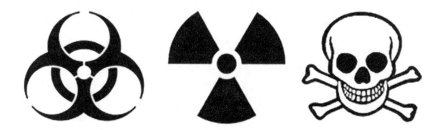

Avoid Unsupported "Medical" Information

Those of us who consider themselves candidates for AD are vulnerable, and often desperate for information, direction, and reassurance. Beware falling into the traps of misinformation and manipulation. Although the web and media can provide volumes of content, there is more bad data than good data out there.

So, when it comes to medical advice, stick with medical school resources or those from government agencies or national organizations like HHS, CDC, AARP, or the Alzheimer's Association (See Resources, Appendix II). Avoid chatrooms and discussion groups unless verifiably sponsored by such organizations. Don't pay attention to advertisements. Turn a blind eye to "breakthroughs" or "associations between [*Fill in the Blank*] and Alzheimer's disease" publicized in any unregulated source, from your inbox to the tabloid rack in the supermarket checkout aisle. Self-treatment with supplements or other unproven therapies, even if harmless, may delay diagnoses and earlier treatment or advance planning.

Beware of "Clinically Shown" or "Clinically Proven" Positive Results

What does "Clinically Proven" Even Mean?

(The following explanation, with which I agree, came from Bard (now Gemini), a large language machine-learning model from Google AI, November 24, 2023).

- - - - - - - - - - - - -

"The phrase 'clinically proven' is often used in marketing and advertising to convey the impression that a product or treatment has been rigorously tested and found to be effective. However, the phrase is not scientifically valid or meaningful; it can be used to describe a wide range of studies, from small and poorly designed to large and well-designed, provides no information about the strength of the evidence, and does not guarantee that a treatment is safe or effective for everyone."

The term "clinical" simply means that something is related to the practice of medicine. Therefore, a "clinically proven" claim could refer to anything from a single case study to a large, randomized controlled trial. In science, something is only considered to be 'proven' if there is overwhelming evidence to support it. In the context of clinical research, this means that there should be multiple, well-designed studies that consistently show the same positive results."

My observation: Although the phrase permeates advertisements for over-the-counter medications in all media, all the time, "clinically proven" appears in the title of just thirty-six of the National Library of Medicine's more than 36 million citations of the published biomedical literature. One could then legitimately argue that "clinically proven" agents (when compared with "scientifically proven" ones) may truly be "one in a million."

Dietary Supplements—What Everyone Needs to Know

From the American Medical Association:[449] While more than 50% of US adults are taking supplements, the AMA is not supportive of their use for curing disease:

- "Supplements are not permitted to be sold as if they prevent or treat disease."
- "The FDA regulates them as a subcategory of food."
- "The manufacturer can introduce anything into the market that they believe is safe."

- "The FDA's job is to identify the products that are causing harm *after* they've been on the market and remove them from store shelves."
- "'Natural' doesn't mean good for you. Cocaine and heroin are natural."
- "Social media can stretch the truth: even the very lax rules around promoting a supplement are being really pushed to the limit."

Look closely for the government-required warning asterisks (*). In advertisements, you will find them in the text with the smallest font, in the most inconspicuous location, somewhere following a prominent assertion like:

"(Xxxxxxxx® is a dietary supplement that has been clinically shown to help with mild memory loss associated with aging.*)"

The first asterisk (*) points to the often hard-to-find second one (*), in a tiny font in print ads and for the briefest of moments onscreen in TV ads:

"*These statements have not been evaluated by the Food and Drug Administration. This product is not intended to diagnose, treat, cure, or prevent any disease."

Unlike the FDA, which approves or disapproves pharmaceuticals, there is no agency monitoring supplement manufacturing, or the consistency or quality of ingredients. Contamination is generally discovered only after people get sick or die.

Specifically, over-the-counter dietary supplements marketed to improve memory and cognitive function have been dangerous as well as ineffective. Unsafe dosages and adulteration with unapproved drugs are common. As an example, *five drugs not approved for human use in the United States were found in cognitive enhancement supplements purchased online.* Drugs detected in samples were not mentioned on the label, while the marketed drugs were often not to be found. Seventy-five percent of product labels describing the *amount* of active drug in the product were inaccurate. Consumers could have been exposed to dosages up to four times greater than recommended, and to as many as four unapproved agents in an individual product.[450] From the Food and Drug Administration: "From 2007 through 2021, 1068 unique dietary supplement products were found to be adulterated with active pharmaceutical ingredients nowhere on the label."[451] The health effects of consuming untested combinations of unapproved drugs at unpredictable dosages without medical or regulatory oversight are unknown.[450]

Prevagen® (apoaequorin: a.k.a. "The Elephant in the Room")

This synthetic protein, copied from the DNA of a glow-in-the-dark jellyfish and produced by fermenting genetically modified bacteria, is the most widely marketed "memory-enhancing" dietary supplement. As of 2020, "Three million people are estimated to have purchased Prevagen® since it was first launched in 2007." (https://www.wired.com/story/prevagen-made-millions-fda-questioned-safety/)

From the manufacturer's website: "Prevagen® is a dietary supplement that has been clinically shown to help with mild memory loss associated with aging.*" (See "What does "Clinically Proven" Even Mean?" on page 180). Their website offers the same FDA-required statement: "*These statements have not been evaluated by the Food and Drug Administration. This product is not intended to diagnose, treat, cure, or prevent any disease."

The Good News:

Apparently, no jellyfish are harmed in the process.

The phrase they market, "mild memory loss associated with aging" is not a disease, nor is it associated with AD brain pathology. It, in fact, refers to "age-related cognitive decline" (ARCD), i.e., "normal for age," or "senior moments."[59] There have been at least seven class-action lawsuits filed in five different states for falsely advertising Prevagen®. The cost to the company of a 2021 settlement that required rebates for Prevagen® purchases was estimated to be tens of millions of dollars.

The Medical Letter on Drugs and Therapeutics, a respected, peer-reviewed, biweekly medical journal with a worldwide circulation in the hundreds of thousands has been evaluating pharmaceuticals since 1959. The conclusion of their 2021 review was: "There is no acceptable evidence that apoaequorin (Prevagen®) is effective for memory improvement. Patients should be advised not to take it."[452]

Expert opinion is against other marketed memory-aid supplements as well. Authors of the most recent (2022) medical textbook on AD, *"Memory Loss, Alzheimer's Disease and Dementia, 3rd Edition,"*[43] do not recommend Vitamin E, B-complex, Gingko biloba, fish oil, Prevagen®, or nonsteroidal anti-inflammatory drugs (NSAIDs) for their patients.[437] Similarly, in their 2018 extensive *Annals of Internal Medicine* review of "Over-the-Counter Supplement Interventions to Prevent Cognitive Decline, Mild Cognitive Impairment, and Clinical Alzheimer-Type Dementia," Butler et al. concluded that "evidence is insufficient to recommend any OTC supplement for cognitive protection in adults with normal cognition or MCI."[453]

Supplements, the placebo response, and superstitious behavior: Why might otherwise reliable health professionals, friends, relatives, and neighbors (as opposed to paid actors or celebrities) swear by supplements—memory-enhancing or otherwise? The "placebo response" refers to an improvement in symptoms after receiving an inactive treatment.[454]

Beneficial placebo effects can be *learned*, resulting from Pavlovian conditioning—the pairing of the inert placebo with a positive effect that the placebo did not cause. Effective placebos include the creation of an expectation. Expectations can come from testimonials, the reassuring effect of white coats, relaxation techniques, distraction, hypnosis, as well as simple encouragement and suggestion (i.e., "You'll just feel a little pressure," or "This is *the good stuff*").

Testimonials and recommendations from celebrities and actors in commercials, well-meaning individuals, disease-specific websites, friends, and family can all contribute to a placebo effect. Placebo responses can reflect other uncontrolled mechanisms, as well, including spontaneous improvement, patient bias, or the many unknowable factors that influence the natural course of a disease. In standard drug studies, placebo responses are seen and accounted for in both experimental and control (a.k.a. "placebo") groups. Positive responses to placebos in drug studies are common and expected, with an average frequency of 35%.[455,456]

A *superstition* is an irrational belief or behavior. The mechanisms that underly the psychology of our superstitions, also contribute to placebo effects. Both placebos and superstitions rely on the pairing of a previously unrelated event or behavior with activation of the brain's reward system. Superstitious behavior comes from the unconsciously "conditioned" tendency to repeat previously neutral actions that are accidentally or randomly rewarded (reinforced) when they happen to occur at the same time as a positive event, like deciding to wear your "lucky" hat because the last two times you wore it, your team won.

How to Play It Safe in the Supplement Aisle

If you're going to try a supplement that has not received FDA approval (i.e., heavily advertised, "herbal," "organic," celebrity-endorsed, "pharmacist recommended," "homeopathic," free sample, "money-back guarantee," coupon, "holistic," "as seen-on-TV," etc., *think twice*. First, continue doing everything your doctor recommends, then discuss any OTC products with your provider before starting. Never substitute these products for prescribed medications.

Consult reliable sources (See Resources, Appendix II): National organizations may have position papers and information for the public often designed to "out" speculations not supported by science. (e.g., The National Institutes of Health/ National Institute on Aging, American Medical Association, Centers for Disease Control and Prevention, the Food and Drug Administration, American Academy of Neurology, AARP, the Alzheimer's Association, your state's health department.) Stick to websites of medical institutions whose names you recognize (and watch for soundalikes): e.g., Mayo Clinic, WebMD, Medscape, Medline Plus (from the National Library of Medicine). Your spam folder is there for a reason.

Do the research: If you're going to try something herbal, holistic, unproven, etc., it's important to keep your provider in the loop. Confirm that what you're taking is what it's claimed to be and is essentially harmless. There's a big difference between science and testimonials.

Even then, "Trust, but Verify!" For example, the very first suggestion that one of my (ex-) doctors offered after delivering a serious diagnosis to me (over the phone) was to encourage me to "subscribe" to a program of two vitamin/mineral supplements "specifically tailored" to my condition. They kindly offered me the use of their own unique "discount code." My research (both in multiple traditional sources and in "Smell Test: The World-Wide Journal of Self-serving Bullshit") found no documented medical reason to buy those products for that condition.

Homeopathic medicines have a devoted following and have been around since the late eighteenth century. Homeopathy is based on two principles far outside the realm of established science: (1) The "Law of Similars" states that one *treats* a symptom with a substance that *causes* that symptom, and (2) the "Law of Infinitesimals" says that drastically diluting that "similar" remedy significantly magnifies its strength. One could argue that, given their extreme dilutions, homeopathic remedies are likely to have few adverse effects. However, the same concerns discussed below regarding contamination, sourcing, substitution, reliability, and safety of herbal products and other OTC preparations apply.

"Herbal" Product Safety:

On the drugstore shelf, one manufacturer's hydroponically grown, meticulously manufactured, organic, plant-based dietary supplement is indistinguishable from another with the identical generic name. A product claiming exactly the same content, on the same shelf, may appear to be a better bargain. However, you have no way to determine where any such item came from or how it was manufactured.

That "same" product could just as easily (and much less expensively) be derived from some unverified weed, harvested from a ditch behind a third-world landfill, and shipped to the States in secondhand fifty-gallon drums previously containing God-knows-what. Potency, quality, consistency, bioavailability, and the potential for dangerous contamination vary tremendously and unpredictably among all such unregulated products.

If your choice is based on published research, be sure of three things: it is published in a legitimate journal, the agent is essentially harmless, and its alleged beneficial effects appear to be supported. If a source is not obviously credible, find someone to assess the original paper for you. After doing the research, take the next step and *trust only the exact formulation* of the non-prescription product used in the study.

An excellent example of "trust only the *exact formulation*" is the "AREDS2" multivitamin supplement endorsed by eye specialists for decades. Its use slows age-related macular degeneration (AMD), the leading cause of blindness in those over age sixty. The *very specific combination* of vitamins, supplements, and their doses that comprises AREDS2 was established as safe and effective in a well-crafted and replicated series of multi-center, randomized, double-blind, placebo-controlled, peer-reviewed clinical trials. Commonly recommended by ophthalmologists, products with the *identical* composition judged helpful in the original trials are sold commercially by multiple reputable companies. (From the *Journal of the American Medical Association*.)[457]

And a much less reassuring and more frequently encountered OTC example of "trust only the exact formulation" . . .

Have you ever heard of "SAW PALMETTO"?

Saw Palmetto is an extract from the plant, *Serenoa repens*. Hundreds of over-the-counter (OTC) versions are widely available. The majority are inexpensive, commonly recommended as "Take Saw Palmetto" by family doctors and urologists and used by millions of men as a non-prescription remedy for symptoms of an enlarged prostate. Like all herbal medicines, palmetto extracts are complex mixtures of organic compounds extracted by diverse chemical and physical means from various parts of the harvested plant material.

All herbals are subject to wide variability: from the site and time at which they are harvested, to the manufacturing procedures and chemicals used to extract the product, and the conditions under which they are grown, transported, and stored. The entire basis of the medical validation behind palmetto extract's wide use comes from a few well-conducted studies employing just one manufacturer's unique preparation. That product, alone, earned approval (by name) from the European Medicines Agency (EMA, the European Union's equivalent of the FDA) as a "well-established medical use product." The EMA's positive evaluation was based on valid published results from—and comparisons with—other palmetto products. This is the only one, out of hundreds of available and identical-looking formulations of saw palmetto extract, deemed "approved" by anyone.

Unfortunately, this unique formulation, specifically the "hexanic lipidosterolic extract" of *Serenoa repens* (marketed as Permixon®), is only produced in France by a single manufacturer. It is licensed and available only in the EU. Permixon® is neither licensed by the FDA, nor available in the US. If you search for this one product by name to try and purchase it online in the US, Google will offer up dozens of other brands of someone else's untested and unapproved palmetto sap.

As of March 2023, seeking "Permixon®" from Amazon. com yielded 853 results. None of them have that brand name, are identified as formulated in the same way, have been tested for safety and efficacy, or are recommended by any regulatory agency. Yet every bottle you can buy, from every source outside Europe, is also "Saw Palmetto." [458,459] One can't help wondering what else on those supermarket and pharmacy shelves is only masquerading as "safe and effective."

In a previous draft of this section, I wrote: "Stick to chain pharmacies; the internet is a dangerous place to buy reliable chemicals and pharmaceuticals." However, a November 2022 National Public Radio story titled "Certain Vapes and Medicines Banned By FDA Are Still Being Sold" casts doubt on chain pharmacies as a reliable neighborhood safety net for non-prescription items. Investigative reporting revealed that items *banned by the FDA* (including cough medicines tied to unexplained infant deaths, and a gummy bear flavored vape decorated with cartoon characters) were "ubiquitous in our daily lives." Their availability in gas stations, mini marts, and chain pharmacies was well documented, and attributed to the limitations of FDA enforcement.[460]

So, sadly, the corner drug store and the internet can both be medical minefields. People lie. "Scientific evidence" is fabricated. Oversight is dimmed and endorsements are unsubstantiated. There is no way to learn the safety and actual composition of products you are buying (or, for that matter, ideas you are buying into). Good luck with that!

Avoid the Lure of New or Unproven Therapies

Most studies of new treatments have been "preliminary," "pilot," "proof of concept," and overall, very limited. A number of potentially viable treatments for AD have been discussed in the scientific and lay press but are not yet ready for "prime time"—i.e., for obtaining an official recommendation by professional societies or regulatory bodies. Keep in mind that in the large, definitive 2017 review by the National Academies ("Preventing Cognitive Decline And Dementia"), the only preventive intervention they found with a risk/benefit ratio that justified advising the public was blood pressure management.[183]

"Metabolic enhancement," also known as "precision medicine," is a recent example of a controversial approach to AD that has been characterized as a "non-validated treatment.[461-466] "Precision medicine" advocates note that while AD depends on many factors, all previous minimally effective interventions have targeted only one metabolic pathway, such as amyloid or tau. The theory of "metabolic enhancement" therapy centers on testing for, identifying, and then simultaneously targeting up to fifty of an individual's unique genetic or biomarker-identified risk factors. It tracks those factors' metabolic pathways, the patterns of which they claim are unique to each patient. "Personalized" treatments consist of diet and lifestyle choices, medications, and supplements.

In their initial results, nine of the first ten patients with various cognitive deficiencies "displayed *subjective* or objective improvement in cognition."[463] However, criticism soon followed, labeling such therapies, for the time being, "non-validated treatments." Daly, et al., writing in the journal *Theoretical Medicine and Bioethics*, cautions about the ethics and risks of "overstating evidence for metabolic enhancement."[467] For any such advance, researcher Gert Helgesson recommends creating a "framework to protect patient interests and avoid decisions driven by the possible benefits to the treating physician, clinic, hospital, or commercial agent."[468]

While some initially non-validated treatments may eventually be shown to work, many more "promising" findings will not. However, the authors, some journal editors, and those seeking to profit from an AD "breakthrough" are always hopeful. Original journal sources usually appropriately reference the need for additional or larger studies, external validation, comparisons with other treatments, and long-term assessments of the magnitude and duration of benefit or the development of harm. News magazines, blog posts, press releases, or advertisements generally skip the same cautions. It is far too early for these novel therapies to have proved themselves worthy of your hope, time, or money. Feel free to browse, but I wouldn't sign up for the treatment or invest in the stock.

There are many other examples of non-validated treatments. You will hear or read about them, often in excitedly optimistic terms. Most, however, are in the early stages, with only very preliminary evidence to present. Currently "under study" in animals or humans, the following examples are in varying stages of development and validation. Risk levels vary widely.[469] They include:

External brain stimulation: "neuromodulation;"[470] "repetitive transcranial alternating current stimulation;"[471] "repetitive transcranial magnetic stimulation" and other variations on electromagnetic fields;[469] "auditory closed-loop stimulation;"[472] "slow-wave activity enhancement" to improve cognition;[473]

"gamma brain-wave stimulation;"[474] "light and sound therapy" (https://www.cognitotx.com); low-intensity brain-focused ultra-sound;[475] and "deep brain stimulation" with surgically implanted neurostimulators.[469]

The "Check My Brain" platform allegedly uses stem cells and the transformation of hairs into neurons to offer: 1) early diagnosis of brain diseases by detecting biomarkers in cell cultures; 2) the ability to measure disease progression through changes in biomarkers levels; and 3) personalized instructions on dietary, supplementary, and other approaches that could potentially benefit an individual's brain.[469]

Exosomes are small, membranous particles discharged bud-like from cell membranes that are believed to allow transport of that cell's characteristics to other cells. The ability of exosomes to deliver RNA sequences across the blood-brain barrier is proposed to one day offer a unique approach to AD.[469]

Irisin: In AD mouse models, increases in Irisin (a hormone that is considered a crucial regulator of the cognitive benefits of exercise) improved both cognitive deficits and neuropathologic changes. Irisin is viewed as a potential therapeutic agent for treating cognitive disorders including AD.[476]

Increasing brain oxygen: Hyperbaric oxygen therapy (HBOT) is a validated medical treatment that involves breathing pure oxygen in a pressurized environment. The increased pressure boosts the amount of oxygen dissolved in the blood and is used to heal tissues and fight infections. HBOT is generally accepted to treat medical conditions like gas gangrene, decompression sickness, carbon monoxide poisoning, severe burns, and non-healing wounds. In a mouse model of AD, HBOT improved cerebral blood flow (CBF) and reduced both the existing volume and new formation of amyloid plaques. Elderly patients with significant memory loss exposed to HBOT for sixty daily sessions over three months had an increase in

CBF and a 16% improvement in memory scores over their baseline test performance.[477]

Other proposed sources of extra brain oxygen are ozone[469] and, in the extreme, omental transplants (surgical transposition of a section of omentum from the abdomen to the brain). Omentum, the extensive and vascular flat layer of fatty tissue that rests on the surface of the abdominal organs, is proposed as a way of increasing the flow of blood and oxygen to delay and even improve the clinical manifestations of AD.[478,479]

Fecal transplants from young to old mice appear to improve aging-induced neurocognitive and immune impairments.[480]

PART IV: A GUIDEBOOK FOR THE JOURNEY

Chapter 6
DEALING WITH TODAY, PREPARING FOR TOMORROW

Like the book itself, this segment begins with the realities and ends with hope: for you, for me, for our loved ones. Chapter 6 is less about telling you what I know and more about what I would consider when deciding what to do for myself or to discuss with a patient, friend, or family member sharing their cognitive concerns. I offer my final thoughts on providers, testing, caregiving, coping with "normal" memory loss and diagnosed dementia, preparing for the worst, and some suggestions for social and political action.

This chapter represents my personal conclusions from a review of what we have learned together, with evidence-based suggestions for both the present and the future. I offer it as a conversation with you, the readers, my aging contemporaries, or those who care about and for us.

At a time of explosive growth in the study of AD and its precursors, we must reconcile the present state of knowledge dealing with memory, cognition, and dementia with what we've learned from summaries by major medical organizations in the last ten years. I'm offering informed suggestions based on what was known before and what transpired since on how to prepare for our future, with what I hope is a clear-eyed look down my road and yours. We all have the same question: *What can I do if my subjective decline and absent-mindedness get worse?*

You and I are not alone. Are you also streaming the second season of your favorite show while trying to remember what the first season was about? Oh, and Amazon just dropped off a package. "What did I order?" I am a member of a large email discussion group made up of dozens of critical care medical specialists worldwide. Many of these doctors, at the height of their professional achievements and responsibilities, literally have our lives in their hands every day. I recall a significant discussion among these worried health professionals sharing their concerns and seeking reassurance from their peers about *their* memory difficulties, which, as described, were likely age-related. The point is that such concerns are universal.

Time for a Reality Check

Currently we have no proof that medicine can offer treatment for the underlying processes of Alzheimer's dementia. Available options can lessen symptoms and "roll back the clock" for a bit. There is a ton of ongoing research, driven by an abundance of brilliant, optimistic, and committed scientists worldwide. There is time, particularly for those mostly young doctors and researchers, to make important findings.

However, disease research can take decades. Aside from making beneficial lifestyle changes (which we should all be doing), in the absence of a cure we need to plan for a future that we may be unable to manage for ourselves. My goal has been to help you through helping myself: "Prepare for the worst and hope for the best."

First Steps for the Worried

What Symptoms Do I Have?
Talk to friends and family. Don't be surprised if those who care about us are already seeking ways to start a discussion. We may hesitate to share our self-identified concerns in case they start

seeing and treating us differently. If you've noticed a problem, the chances are that others have, as well. Sharing this book and talking about one's issues can only advance communication and understanding. Failure to plan for all possibilities will make it harder for everyone. Add their impressions to yours to more clearly define the changes you perceive. It is particularly important to distinguish between failing *memory* and problems with *cognition* (chapter 1).

What Are My Risk Factors? (See table 2, chapter 4.)

Work on these, no matter what. Use your cognitive concerns as one more motivator to make those positive lifestyle changes that we all put off. Fortunately, they can be beneficial at any age (See "Prevention" in Chapter 4). Just as fear of cancer may trigger finally stopping smoking, memory loss plus fear of AD should provide similar motivation to clean up one's act.

When to Seek Medical Attention for Your Memory

We all make excuses for memory lapses in ourselves and others. Eventually we come across one of those scary "10 Warning Signs" lists in an advertisement, a newsfeed, a magazine cover, or from the guest doctor on your local news channel. No matter how you get there, the realization that you or a loved one is having a "memory problem" should be enough to generate a visit to a primary care provider.

Examples of early signs and symptoms (from Reliable Sources):

Alzheimer's Association: "10 Early Signs and Symptoms of Alzheimer's," https://www.alz.org/alzheimers-dementia/10 _signs: [481]

- Memory loss that disrupts daily life
- Challenges in planning or solving problems
- Difficulty completing familiar tasks
- Confusion with time or place
- Trouble understanding visual images and spatial relationships
- New problems with words in speaking or writing
- Misplacing things and losing the ability to retrace steps
- Poor or decreased judgment
- Withdrawal from work or social activities
- Changes in mood and personality

AARP: Repetition and getting lost are two signs from AARP's "Seven Early Warning Signs of Dementia You Shouldn't Ignore" that can be added to those above. https://www.aarp .org/caregiving/health/info-2019/dementia-warning-signs .html[482]

Some other signs can be:

- Getting angry with yourself
- Frustration during conversations with those close to you
- Conflicts based on memory failings
- You find family or friends:
  - adding things to your list of daily reminders
  - finishing your sentences while you are still searching for a word
  - correcting your recollections, filling in the blanks
- You are impacting others:
  - being late
  - getting "a little turned around"
  - dropping tasks, from forgetting to pick up milk on the way home, to forgetting to pick up a child at a recurring after-school event

You May Already Know When It's Time to Get Checked Out

If you suspect you're not "right," there's a fair chance you are correct. You will spot the earliest clues to the possibility of cognitive decline and will likely feel that something is wrong well before an office exam or standard neuropsychological tests show an abnormality. The sense of things "not being right" that precedes a diagnosis of Subjective Cognitive Decline (SCD, chapter 2) can be the earliest symptom of AD.

Like every symptom, there are multiple possible causes: from medical conditions to substance use to stress. Think of your personal doubts as a sensitive (but not specific) test you are performing on yourself. Compare the present with the past as only you can do. Use any subtle changes as motivation for finally adopting those wellness goals on your to-do list, simple changes that can slow both physical and cognitive aging.

> Been there! "Normal for age" in two eminent neurologists' offices, but still not satisfied, so I researched this book. We're not always correct, but until we are a lot farther down this road, we know ourselves better than our doctors do.

Look for "Red Flags"

Personal issues or past events that increase our vulnerability to AD include:

- Having a family member (parent, child, or sibling) with dementia puts you at risk. Any family history of AD increases one's chance of AD by two to four times (chapter 4).

- Recent emergency department visits and hospitalization for *any* reason can precipitate cognitive decline. Hospitals are among the many stressors that, when superimposed on age- and illness-related declines in physiologic reserve, can serve as a tipping point.[483]
- Memory lapses are becoming frequent enough or sufficiently noticeable to concern you, friends, or a family member.[24]
- Changing speech patterns are recognizable in early stages. These may be subtle and most obvious to those who know a person well.[237] An increased use of pronouns may be interfering with communication (chapter 4).
- Cognitive decline can masquerade as hearing loss (and vice versa), another common problem with the elderly.
- Depression or mood change.
- Altered handwriting is one of the earliest noticeable signs of Alzheimer's disease.[253]
- Naming difficulty and the tip-of-the-tongue phenomenon for proper nouns are clues.[129] (Like the Google search I did for ["actor + pilot + island +beach + ball"] to extract Tom Hanks's name from the tip of *my* tongue.)
- Getting lost or "turned around." Ending up at one familiar destination when headed for another.
- Running out of Post-It® notes or finding them in unexpected locations.

What to Expect from Your Primary Care Provider

Most of us should start there. They should know you and may either be able put your mind at rest early or confirm some changes you can pursue together. You are seeking reassurance, consideration of all possible causes for your symptoms, and a plan for evaluation, management and follow-up.

Start with the provider who knows you best (second to you, of course—*you* are the one who truly knows you best). If it still doesn't feel right, keep looking for a primary care provider. You might also consider working with a geriatric specialist. These physicians see only older patients, day-after-day, perhaps with added experience, insights, time to spend, and age-specific resources to call on.

Take someone with you who knows you well and can describe what they and others see. That person's observations can only improve your provider's understanding (and may teach you a thing or two). Give them some time alone with the doctor so they can speak more freely.

> Going alone to talk about your memory with a doctor is about as useful as bringing your high school yearbook to a job interview.

Routine Good Medical Practice Dictates (likely over more than one appointment):

A thorough history of your symptoms, including what friends and family say they notice. A review of your medical and family history, and medications. The doctor will ask a lot of questions about your memory, including: How long have you or others noticed a problem? What sorts of things are the most difficult to remember? Did symptoms come on gradually or suddenly? Are you having trouble with routine daily tasks? The provider will also want to know how you've been eating and sleeping, whether you've been depressed or stressed lately, and generally about what's been happening in your life. There should be an assessment of the status of your ongoing medical problems, their treatment, and a discussion of their status, prognosis, and possible contribution to your memory concerns. Maybe keep a log in advance of the appointment. Be clear in stating your questions and concerns; write them out in advance.

Consideration of other medical diagnoses that could be causing your symptoms. A physical examination matched to your level of general health, and likely laboratory work relevant to the above.

A mental status evaluation: The most common are the mini-mental status examination (MMSE), and the clock drawing test. Those and other brief screening tests (chapter 4) can be administered in five to ten minutes and can accurately diagnose dementia, but not the earlier stages of cognitive decline. Those still suspected of dementia or MCI who pass the screen can be referred for the full standard battery of neuropsychological tests.

What to Expect from a Memory Specialist

As you progress in your search for answers, you may see a memory specialist for a consultation. This category of specialist includes physician neurologists or psychologists (specifically, neuropsychologists). These doctors specialize in disorders of the brain and nervous system, preferably with a special interest in memory problems. The basics of any specialist consultation would include a discussion of your neurological concerns in depth, along with medical, family, and medication history.

Testing, including a more involved neurological and mental status exam, could potentially confirm a diagnosis, but more commonly establishes a baseline for ongoing monitoring. Remember that such tests (along with an experienced practitioner's "gestalt") can be specific for MCI and are not sensitive enough to confirm earlier forms of cognitive decline.

Additional advanced neuropsychological testing can distinguish abnormal cognitive performance from normal aging. It does so by testing your various cognitive domains and comparing your scores with the norms for specific age groups. After evaluation, you are entitled to a clear and jargon-free explanation of the findings, their implications, and a plan. Often you will be reassured and booked for a re-evaluation. Less frequently, you will undergo advanced testing of body fluids or brain imaging to more specifically confirm or dismiss the possibility of a diagnosis of AD.[47]

Neurocognitive and Genetic Testing: Yes or No?

Screening for cognitive impairment with neurocognitive testing: In 2020, the US Preventive Services Task Force (USPTF) concluded that "several brief screening instruments can adequately detect cognitive impairment, especially in populations with a higher prevalence of underlying dementia. There is no empiric evidence, however, that screening for cognitive impairment or its early diagnosis improves patient, caregiver, family, or clinician decision-making or other important outcomes, nor causes harm."[389]

Screening tests are described in chapter 4. Most can be administered by your provider in ten minutes or less. Understand that preclinical AD and SCD are not detectable by the usual in-office testing, and "normal for age" still includes both of those possibilities.

On the other hand, frank dementia is readily diagnosed by brief, in-office mental status exams (and often first by friends and family members). The diagnosis of MCI requires a comprehensive neuropsychological examination, which typically involves a referral from your provider and hours of testing across multiple cognitive domains.[484]

The threshold for ordering such evaluations differs among providers, varying with multiple factors that include your insurance, their history with and knowledge of you, their comfort and experience with issues of cognitive decline, and their overall impressions.

Any one neuropsychological screening test showing some degree of cognitive impairment is enough to presumptively diagnose MCI (See Chapter 3). However, in most cases, a positive screening test should be followed with the full standard battery of tests to further define specific deficits and serve as a baseline for the road ahead.

Should I Screen Myself for Cognitive Impairment?

The Self-Administered Gerocognitive Exam (SAGE) questionnaire is better than the MMSE in differentiating those with cognitive impairment from normal subjects (i.e., in diagnosing MCI and its progression).[145,146,485] Best of all, it's free at (https://wexnermedical.osu.edu/brain-spine-neuro/memory-disorders/sage). However, self-testing is not for everyone. I don't advise it for those without the resources to follow through with a qualified specialist to interpret the results, place the findings in a broader context, and develop a plan going forward. I strongly recommend discussing self-testing and the USPTF findings with your provider if you're planning on going down that rabbit hole on your own.

Biomarker Testing

If the search for Alzheimer's disease was a TV crime drama, biomarkers would be the fingerprint or DNA evidence that unravels the mystery of "whodunit." Even in the absence of any other indication, the identification of biomarkers *is Alzheimer's disease* in its "preclinical" stage.

Easier and More Frequent Testing Is Coming

As blood tests become more accurate, available, and affordable, busy providers may add biomarkers to their "routine" testing. Unfortunately, they can fail to consider an individual's likely response to a *positive* test. Most doctors love testing because it lessens their risk of missing a diagnosis. After a certain age, or for those with active medical problems, "routine" diagnostic studies become an important part of general medical practice. These include wellness assessments, screening for serious occult disease like common cancers, and "preventive maintenance" like assessing for and monitoring diabetes and elevated cholesterol.

> But biomarker testing is not just "another trip to the lab."
> Before signing on for one of these particular
> tests, ask yourself:
> "How Would a Positive Result Change My Life?"

The Current Understanding of AD and Testing

AD is presently accepted as a continuum along which patients experience a lengthy (preclinical) phase without symptoms. While neuropathological changes are accumulating, cognitive abilities remain normal. Next is a symptomatic phase of progressive cognitive decline without dementia, followed by the onset of functional loss.[198]

Brain changes culminating in dementia begin to accumulate approximately twenty years before clinical signs appear,[53] and biomarker evidence can be detected well before the onset of any symptoms. Most importantly: for the majority of the estimated 47 million people below age seventy who are in that preclinical phase of AD, *a positive test does not mean that the person will inevitably develop clinical disease, and a negative test is not 100% good news.* False negatives occur with every medical test, and as many as one-third of those who clinically suffer from AD have negative scans.[191]

Issues Surrounding Biomarker Testing and Disclosure

Timing: In the current environment, early diagnosis is most often spoken of as "potentially" beneficial. Instead of "early," some emphasize the notion of a "timely" diagnosis, when cognitive and other changes begin to affect patients' lives and the lives of people close to them. Ethnic and cultural groups may vary both in seeking a diagnosis and in their receptiveness to it.[486]

The impact of disclosing positive test results: Expectations play a role. In one study, scans were obtained to identify AD in patients with a previously unclear diagnosis. When results were in line with the care partner's perceptions of the patient's condition (i.e., a positive scan for a patient with signs of cognitive impairment), care partners reported a lack of surprise and a feeling of relief, rather than shock or frustration. When a patient with only mild cognitive impairment received a positive scan result, care partners expressed anxiety.[191]

Perspectives of those who receive disclosure will vary. One asymptomatic neuroscientist who had a negative screening scan as a subject in a research study said that, had the scan been positive, it would have changed his life forever: "I will wake up every morning and wonder whether . . . this is the day I am going to forget something."[191]

As is true with other serious neurodegenerative diseases (like ALS: Amyotrophic Lateral Sclerosis a.k.a. "Lou Gehrig's disease") the benefit of presymptomatic biomarker testing is limited by the absence of preventative treatments to offer, and the inability to predict when (*or even if*) someone who is biomarker positive will develop AD.

Advantages attributed to biomarker testing:[198] Negative biomarker testing can exclude AD and promote the search for other causes of cognitive impairment that are not yet evident clinically. Conversely, when positive, such tests reduce the impact of a delayed diagnosis or misdiagnosis. An early diagnosis when worried patients first seek help for changes in cognition, behavior, or function, may have advantages, even without treatments to reverse the disease. The answer may be important to family members, particularly if there are concerns about genetically mediated early onset AD.

Opportunities do exist for implementing coordinated care plans, improving symptom management, and assuring patient safety. Physicians can address specific issues like anxiety or impaired sleep, and manage medications prescribed for other conditions that may aggravate AD symptoms.

For those who want to explore every option, there is no shortage of clinical trials assessing new therapies. Many of these will require biomarker testing as a condition of enrollment. The earlier the diagnosis, the better the chances for access to trials. "We do not wait until symptoms appear for diseases like cancer, HIV, or osteoporosis. Why should we wait for cognitive impairment to do what we can for AD?"[191]

A positive test can stimulate getting one's affairs in order and planning for the future.[487] Patients may also have an opportunity to consider advance care plans, make end-of-life decisions, alter unhealthy lifestyles, and seek optimal and coordinated medical care. A well-informed patient and family are less likely to end up in crisis situations or premature institutionalization, potentially eliminating those stresses and costs.

Disadvantages attributed to biomarker testing:[191,198] While some widely studied markers can be supportive of a diagnosis of AD, they are not yet recommended for routine diagnostic purposes.[488] Outside of a research setting, few authors recommend biomarker testing in relatively asymptomatic elderly individuals. Up to 73% of those who test positive for biomarkers will *not* develop dementia during their lifetimes, nor can progression be predicted for any individual worried senior.

Knowing the odds is a poor aid to individual decision-making and can add more stress than comfort. Positive results can promote distressing degrees of anxiety and uncertainty in the face of a life-altering diagnosis.

The neurologist or primary care provider who orders biomarker testing on patients with purely subjective concerns may acquire a growing number of diverse elderly patients. All of them will be waiting for the other shoe to drop, while the physician is unable to answer the most relevant questions and has little to offer during this period of unfolding events. Like all diagnostic tests, biomarkers vary in their invasiveness (i.e., "discomfort"), cost, availability, and importantly, accuracy (the ability of a positive test to predict disease, and a negative test to *definitively* rule it out).

Unfortunately, the most accurate biomarker tests are also "invasive" requiring the patient to undergo a lumbar puncture (LP) to obtain a sample of cerebrospinal fluid (chapter 4). Despite their difficulties, the high negative predictive value of such invasive tests makes them the best at definitively *excluding* AD. This ability to accurately identify those who *do not have AD* makes their optimal clinical use to strongly reassure those with some other negative, but less specific, and thus, less reassuring, biomarkers.[72] Better blood tests are coming.

Any potential benefits of biomarkers are yet to be realized. In the absence of effective AD therapies, there appears to be no

advantage to identifying preclinical AD patients for early intervention.[192] Nor can one can predict the time lapse between identifying
an early stage of Alzheimer's and the actual onset of dementia.

One Mayo Clinic neurologist candidly told a *New York Times*
reporter: "[N]ot everyone does progress. Even when they do, it can
be years before there are symptoms. Outside of research studies,
we do not do [definitive and diagnostic] *amyloid scans on clinically normal people because we don't know what to tell them* [emphasis added]."[187]

However, a diagnosis before the onset of cognitive impairment *would change the lives* of millions of adult patients and their
families. Even though the majority will not progress to cognitive impairment, the diagnosis alone will alter one's self-perception and the way they are viewed by those around them.
Families, in addition to concerns for their loved one and the
personal risks and burdens of becoming a long-term caregiver,
are also affected by what a positive result may imply about their
own potential AD risk.[191] It is difficult for anyone to plan and
allocate finite resources for an uncertain future of decline.

It seems to me that since the risk of AD increases with age,
someone with only subjective symptoms and an early
positive biomarker is condemned to a cycle of near-continuous worry. What lies ahead? Repeated (and possibly
more invasive) tests await until cognitive tests become
positive (MCI) and signs of dementia appear (AD), or other
vulnerabilities of aging take over.

Here's the question: Who does early diagnosis actually
benefit?

"TMI" ("Too Much Information"): One goal of screening and disclosure is to offer knowledge that will be helpful for
decision-making as the future unfolds. The challenges presented

to asymptomatic, but biomarker-positive, patients and their families in processing all that information are described as overwhelming—like drinking from a fire hose. It can be helpful to plan for updated discussions as new questions, information, or symptoms emerge. As one cognitive health researcher noted: it is a "whole lot to tell people . . . in a single session, all we *think* we know about Alzheimer's disease."[191]

Other Consequences of Testing

Insurance: While health insurers are prohibited by law from denying coverage for Alzheimer's disease, there is nothing to prevent those writing long-term-care policies and life insurance from refusing to offer a policy to someone who is positive for an AD biomarker.[487]

Health equity is a very real concern. Potentially beneficial supports and interventions are not available to all.

Quality of life: Persons aware of their diagnostic label (either MCI or AD), and its prognosis) report a lower quality of life than those unaware of these facts about themself. The associated sense of loss is unrelated to the actual severity of the cognitive impairment.[489]

Public health risks associated with overdiagnosis:[191] *Nearly 75% with preclinical disease will not progress to clinical AD in their lifetime.* Any shift (numerically, societally, and ethically) from treating those with clinical disease to treating the much larger number with preclinical AD would generate considerable adverse public health consequences. Overdiagnosis, would expose asymptomatic patients to the risks and costs of intervention without the benefit of dementia prevention. There are multiple pathways to dementia, and a large percentage of cognitive decline is *not* attributable to AD. (See Differential Diagnosis: What Else Could It Be? in chapter 4.)

Cost: The societal costs of screening for and treating preclinical AD would be enormous. Informal calculations found that treating half of the 38 million people who have amyloidosis with current standard therapies at $6,000/year would cost $115 billion. (Treating them with 2022-approved Lecanemab at $26,500/year would bring the total to over $500 billion.)

The *nature* of "treatment" will change as large numbers of asymptomatic individuals with positive biomarkers are added to the population under consideration for therapy. The evaluation of such early intervention would have to include factors such as treatment efficacy, side effects and harm, the rate of false positives, and the rate of patient discontinuation of therapy.[191]

> All of this, and still no "disease-modifying therapy." At best, there is a chance of "turning back the clock on memory loss" for six months.

Bioethical Considerations

Preclinical Biomarker Testing in Research and Disclosure of Results[191,486]

When asymptomatic individuals enroll as subjects in research studies, they often undergo biomarker testing. For participation, it is required that their biomarker status be known. The process of identifying and recruiting presymptomatic individuals for research can include discovering and delivering previously unknown and highly distressing news.[490] Researchers may not be on firm ethical ground if they randomly choose some people to be told their biomarker status and others not to be given that information. Concerns include the risks of known negative reactions to disclosure, including clinical depression, anxiety, and suicide.[191]

Because of the ethical challenges of studying reactions to such disclosures, evidence has come almost exclusively from interventional trials. Those use volunteers who undergo bio-marker testing to determine their status *before* enrollment. This is done to ensure that all those in a studied group share the same AD status.

Remember the asymptomatic neuroscientist study volunteer described earlier who, with a positive test, would have awakened every morning and wondered, "Is this the day I'm going to forget something?" Joining a clinical study is admirable, and a valid option for some patients. Just be sure that you are getting the full spectrum of unbiased pros and cons before undergoing biomarker testing for research purposes.

In one such study, cognitively unimpaired participants with a biomarker result suggesting preclinical AD were no more likely than those with a normal result to experience suicidal thoughts, depression, or anxiety. However, an abnormal result *was* associated with intrusive thoughts and mild distress. Individuals also adjusted their perceived risk of developing AD based on their results.[191]

The individual patient is in the best position to decide what information they should receive after testing. Patient involvement in research requires their consent and the capacity to make their own decisions to participate. Family members, however, are also affected by preclinical diagnoses, may have their own opinions about disclosure, and should be included in discussions surrounding research participation.

Privacy: HIPPAA is the collection of federal rules for healthcare providers and health systems that govern the confidentiality of medical information. Patient confidentiality is a cornerstone of the doctor-patient relationship, and a diagnosis of dementia is a momentous one for close family members. After all, they are likely to eventually take on a significant caring role and will need appropriate information and support to do so. For these reasons, professionals who must reveal a diagnosis of dementia should actively encourage their patients to share this information with their families. If the patient insists on discretion from the doctor, their wish must be honored as long as they are considered capable of making this decision. However, the medical professional may advise that eventually it will be in the patient's best interest to share the truth with loved ones.

Coping with Failing Memory without a Diagnosis

Based on the issues discussed above, not everyone should or will decide to be tested. It is highly likely that your medical consultant will reassure you that your memory lapses are "normal at your age." Good news!

That leaves you with the dilemma of minimizing potential embarrassments at work, family gatherings, or when—once again—you're asking, "Has anyone seen my keys?"

What You Can Do—Now
Clean up your act! (If not now, when?)

- Make a clear-eyed assessment of your overall health and wellness.
- Commit to the healthy lifestyle modifications mentioned frequently above.

- Reducing your risk factors (chapter 4) is never a bad idea.

Consider memory and cognitive training: At the point at which we start to mind (or others start to notice) our "age-related cognitive decline" it may be time to consider "memory training." (Think of it as the grownup version of grade school mnemonics.) While not clearly shown to delay or prevent AD,[182,183,433] "cognitive training" in problem solving, memory, and speed of information processing (often via computer) can improve some long-term cognitive functions and allow those with "normal for age" cognitive failings (ARCD) to continue performing daily activities independently.

Tricks to improve memory have been used by students, teachers, and politicians since the orators of ancient Rome and Greece were memorizing their speeches. There are plenty of sources available. (Amazon.com returned 858 titles when searching for "memory training for adults" in November 2022). Mnemonic strategies (the study of systems to improve memory) are offered for every purpose: from maximizing SAT scores, to avoiding social awkwardness at re-introductions, to winning at card games!

The "memory palace" or "method of loci" is one such effective method. It works by visualizing items to be recalled as occupying a specific physical location within a mental map of a place you know well (home, office, etc.). For recall, you walk through your palace and visualize the items you have "placed" there. The more vivid and detailed the images, the easier they are to remember.

Of course, the usual cautions regarding scams and identity theft apply to any memory training activity that involves a third party. These would be "institutes" or similar-sounding organizations you have never heard of, or individuals or sites offering supplements, website memberships, a subscription you can "cancel any time," or any other almost-too-good-to-be-true proposed solution to forgetting why you went to the store. Think twice about anything that costs more than a paperback book on memory strategies.

Take some comfort: I found it encouraging during my research to discover some reassuring references regarding the inability to remember the word at the tip of the tongue (TOT). Logically, some authors (including at least one I have consulted as a patient) point out that if you can eventually remember the proper noun you were unable retrieve earlier, it means that *it isn't gone*. Instead of experiencing memory *loss*, you are demonstrating the age-related problem of memory *retrieval or recollection*. Your brain cells and the pathways connecting them may be aging, but they have not yet been erased by little bundles of amyloid and tau proteins. The first solid research to support this encouraging theory employed functional MRI images to identify the brain areas involved with TOT as *separate* from those areas associated with *memory failure*.[491]

Coping with "Normal" Aging (as defined and described in chapter 1)

Remember: The largest percentage of us will *not* progress to Alzheimer's. The estimated lifetime risk of Alzheimer's dementia at age forty-five is approximately 1 in 5 (20%) for women and 1 in 10 (10%) for men.[227]

Cope by trying. See what works for you. For me—with some word-finding difficulty—what works is writing, texting, and emailing in lieu of phone calls. I also prefer notes or scripts for speaking, rather than speaking spontaneously, or "off the cuff."

Some valuable public speaking strategies for those with word-finding struggles come from a family member, who is also my favorite medical educator, actor, and off-Broadway producer:

"Think first, then speak. Practice talking more slowly. Pause for effect. Use your hands to take the focus away from your face (and speech) as you search for a word. Use physical redirection by pairing pauses with hand gestures. When taking questions, gain some time with: 'Yes, that question reminds me' . . . or ask the person to repeat the question 'for the audience.'"

Remain positive. You can't live your life making negative predictions for yourself. Embrace the Serenity Prayer. Develop supports early (social interaction, group activities, sports, exercise, yoga, friends, hobbies, mindfulness). Be willing to share your concerns with friends. This is what we *all* worry about. Everyone over sixty will have senior moments. Remember:

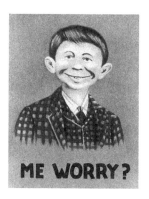

Use all the tools that the modern world provides to minimize forgetting and the awkwardness and discomfort it can bring:

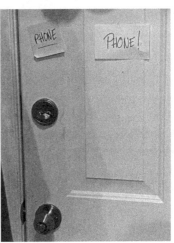

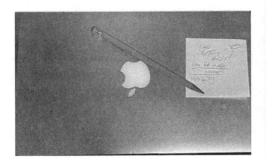

Some of my favorites are low-tech: Post-its®, plus pads and pencils scattered throughout the house. Smartphones never forget (alarms, notes, reminders, and dictation/recording apps). I also can't live without the memo website that sends me email or text reminders at my requested dates, times, and frequency. Voice assistants have rarely let me down, and when they get it wrong, it's at least usually funny.

In my writing, I rely so heavily on the "synonyms" feature of Microsoft Word that I consider Peter Mark Roget (of *Roget's Thesaurus of English Words and Phrases,* 1805) a co-author. I am reminded of comedian Steven Wright's one-liner: "What's another word for thesaurus?"

Consider adding Artificial Intelligence (AI) to your online search techniques. For this, I have been using free versions of commonly available internet AI "assistants." Instead of pages of pay-for-placement links and thousands of web options, AI usually returns a cogent page that answers the question. As a check, I always query more than one, and frequently ask for "up-to-date references," so that I can review their "thinking" myself if I choose to. "Intelligent" or not, always avoid sharing your private information or asking your new best (online) friend for personal, medical, or financial advice. As a minimum, AI can be the quickest road to an answer. Worst case, you've wasted less than a second.

Work: If you have a rewarding job with social and cognitive stimulation, you might do better by cutting back, rather than retiring. Trade your job for volunteer or consulting opportunities.

Be realistic and learn to live with some degree of uncertainty. There is nothing definite in life—it's all about odds and percentages.

"Hope for the best, prepare for the worst." And if you can resist the lure of their commercials, skip the brain supplements. (See chapter 5.)

Find someone to talk to when reassurance and "normal for age" just aren't convincing you or those who care about you. If you think you're declining, admit it to yourself and open an ongoing conversation with family, close friends, your spiritual advisor, a mental health professional, and your physician. Good friends can offer objectivity when you "just don't feel like yourself." A problem for those of us at an early and unclear stage of memory loss or confusion is that we have little access to forums or persons with whom to engage. There are few with whom we can share our intensely personal experiences of memory loss or confusion.

Advice to friends and family: If you see something. . .

Take a page from the Homeland Security playbook: "If you see something, say something!" Denial or the natural inability to recognize gradual cognitive changes in ourselves or those close to us can have later consequences. If early identification is important, those we see less often may more readily exhibit or detect changes that have occurred between contacts. At those infrequent holiday get-togethers, we easily ask each other less important questions, like "Have you lost weight?" or "Is that a new hairstyle?" Yet, there is a tendency to avoid more difficult subjects that might prompt a sudden awareness or validate unspoken concerns. A typical question might be: "Why are your medicines scattered all over the house?" or "How long has Uncle Kenny been wearing his socks inside out?"

You're the one reading the book! Take charge! It's hard to point out to others what they may choose to assume (or hope) is a "natural" absentmindedness in themselves. If you're in the position of seeing symptoms of hesitation or confusion, take the next step and say something. You may be surprised at how often the person is already aware, has been rationalizing growing unease, and is wondering how receptive they would be if confronted with an observer's concerns.

Suspicion of a loved one's cognitive deterioration should trigger a broader discussion among family, friends, and health-care providers. Even early cognitive decline can be dangerous: fraud, medication misadventures, accidents, delayed diagnosis of a treatable medical condition, etc. "If you see something, say something!"

We Should Start Our Own Support Groups!

An internet search confirms abundant options for family members and caregivers of dementia patients to gather and share. However, when seeking such support for those of us just stepping up to that precipice, none of the search results that returned included the word "patient." A conversation with the outreach director at a major medical school's five-star memory center confirmed the wide availability of "support groups for family, partners and caregivers, but none for patients themselves."

How do you drive yourself to an Alzheimer's disease support group and raise your hand for help with trivial problems like finding your glasses or remembering a name? We all have same-age friends. Do we share our experiences and apprehensions with them? I confess—I haven't. Beyond the little jokes we make about "senior moments," like showing up on the wrong day, I suspect most of us WWW's ("Worried Well or Worse") don't even talk to our spouses about the extent of our symptoms and fears. There is a need for such WWW groups. Find one or start one. Tell your friends. Refer to this book. It all helps.

When to Doubt "The Experts"

When should the mixture of anecdote, gut feeling, and irrational fear rise to challenge the acknowledged superiority of doctors and their science? It will vary with the patients and their loved ones, and with their preconceptions, values, and expectations. Don't discount your gut feelings about those you've known so well for so long. Keep them safe, no matter how "normal" they were the last time they spent twenty minutes with their busy doctor. "Normal for age" at its most basic level is not a Band-Aid we seek from the medical profession and their tests. For the most part, like pornography or bullshit, we know "normal for age" when we observe it. We have seen it around us our entire lives: Grandpa's repetitive war stories, the final life trajectories of our parents' friends, then our family members, and now our contemporaries, colleagues, and former classmates. If you, like me, are still worried after being told you're OK, you might want to reread chapter 2 on "subjective cognitive decline."

"Sometimes, the only cure for someone who insists that they are ill is to take them at their word."[492]

I still don't know for certain if I'm the one who's right, or if it's the two eminent neurologists who released me back into the stream of "worried well" overflowing the basements of their ivory towers, Post-its® in hand. If what you need is reassurance, take it and go on. I try not to be too critical of those who appear to whitewash the gravity of my latest lost objects or memories with: "Hey, it's normal at your age."

Reassurance is a timeless palliative approach that began with Hippocrates. I have often used it myself with patients, family, and friends to ease concerns, particularly when there is not much anyone can do. When reassurance is all you have as a provider, it is a lot better than nothing.

Dealing with a "Likely Alzheimer's" Diagnosis

Talking to Your Provider

If you're going to meet with your medical provider, take someone with you. Ask how sure the doctor is regarding your diagnosis. What specific factors influenced the conclusion about your mental acuity? What about a second opinion? A specialist? An academic center? What are the chances of a false positive test? Do you need a repeat or another confirmatory test?

Review the likelihood of an inherited factor and consider suggestions regarding family testing. Inquire about the other dementias or neurological syndromes in the differential diagnosis (chapter 4) and satisfy yourself that your doctor has considered them and ruled them out. AD is by far the most common, but some of the others may have treatments or different implications for family members.

Talking to Your Family About an Alzheimer's Diagnosis[493]

How do you tell someone you love about *their* diagnosis? Why would we even tell someone they have or are likely to develop AD? The answer: because you respect them. Allow your loved one to preserve autonomy in decision-making about future care and treatment for as long as possible. Issues surrounding day-to-day finances and accounts, as well as long-term wishes, need to be explored. Many already recognize that "something is not right."

Be honest and clear. Use the difficult words. Knowing can bring some relief. Answering remaining questions, providing reliable information sources, and formulating plans can be reassuring.

Bring backup: friends, clergy, consultants, therapists, extended family, support groups. Ideally, have the conversation with your loved one's health care provider for explanations and input on diagnosis, treatment, follow-up, and care. Tailor the conversation to their level of understanding. Don't go into overload unless the patient asks for more. Stay positive, be present, supportive, and "in the moment." Let them know that you will be there for them.

Telling loved ones about your own Alzheimer's diagnosis: First, be sure about the basic information before sitting down for such a challenging conversation. Plan for what you will say. Choose a comfortable place or situation that has positive memories or good vibes. Include a discussion about future care options and the likely increasing need for support of all kinds.

That's a lot to absorb, so stop and allow space for acceptance, followed by questions. If you doubt your ability to convey both the personal and medical aspects of such a discussion, you could bring the meeting to your physician, or write it down and go over it with your doctor or a trusted friend or family members who fully understands your situation and supports your choices.

To the Reader: Take Care of Yourself

Regardless of your relationship to the patient (self, family, friend, caregiver): access a support community and maintain regular connections with friends and family. Exercise. Adopt mindfulness and stress-reduction techniques. Seek quality information and keep up with the latest via reliable sources (Alzheimer's Association, AARP, National Institute of Aging, Alzheimers.gov, your local Area Agency on Aging. See Appendix II—Resources.)

Ask for help when you need it.

Genetic Testing (See chapter 4)

Genetic testing is an important decision for both patients and family members (who should be given their own opportunity to decide, in consultation with *their* physician and, potentially, a genetic counselor). Testing for APOE4, the most powerful risk gene for AD, is readily available, even online and by mail, but "not recommended for the assessment of future risk because

APOE lacks sufficient predictive value at the individual level." Many normal elderly carry an APOE allele, and many AD patients do not."[65]

Genetic testing should clearly be a "yes" when the concern is *early-onset* AD. Since testing is most useful when neurological disorders are caused by alterations in one specific gene, testing those whose parents or grandparents developed Alzheimer's before age sixty-five can reveal their risk of carrying the gene and passing it on to their children. (Early onset Parkinson's disease also falls into the single-gene category).

However, genetic testing is not for everyone. Even though inheriting APOE4 neither defines the presence of AD nor indicates any particular stage,[49] just the knowledge of one's APOE4 status can negatively influence behavior, as well as both objective and subjective cognition.[61] Along with some quantifiable increased genetic risk for AD, asymptomatic carriers, who may have witnessed family members decline, can develop a heightened awareness of their own thinking, be more concerned about cognitive function, and wind up labelled as having subjective cognitive decline (chapter 2) with the additional worry *that* entails. Most patients can simply be advised of the modest increased risk of AD in first-degree relatives of AD patients, and that age of onset tends to be similar in families.

Genetic research in AD is ongoing. New information appears constantly (at various levels of certainty and acceptance), so check back periodically with your original sources of information. Regardless of whether one chooses to test or not, genetic counselors may be the most knowledgeable consultants for family concerns. You should be able to get a referral from your memory specialist. Children's hospitals are often well staffed in this area, and the American Board of Genetic Counseling and the National Society of Genetic Counselors provide searchable online directories of genetic counselors worldwide.

Maximizing Outcomes after a Diagnosis

Optimize General Health

Everything in this section also applies equally to those who are not facing an AD diagnosis but want to improve their general well-being and cognitive health.

Wellness measures as recommended by The Institute of Medicine and World Health Organization are beneficial to everyone. To reduce risks of cognitive and physical decline with aging, individuals should: be physically active; reduce and manage cardiovascular risk factors (including hypertension, diabetes, obesity, and smoking); regularly discuss and review health conditions and medications that might influence cognitive health with a health-care professional; follow a Mediterranean diet; and reduce or cease harmful substance use.[5,180] (See Risk Reduction, chapter 4.)

For the greatest benefit, go with wellness ASAP. Start getting the whole person in shape now, rather than taking pills for "this and that" later. To quote a ninety-two-year-old dementia patient speaking to his grandson (a National Public Radio producer) in 2021: *"My God. If I had known I was going to live this long, I would've taken better care of myself."*

Address all medical issues. Don't miss something preventable or treatable. Sensory impairments (hearing and vision loss) are widespread among older adults and frequently contribute to concerns about cognition. Since all standard cognitive tests depend heavily on intact hearing and vision, sensory impairment can render cognitive evaluations unreliable or even invalid.[14] Those with sensory loss have statistically faster rates of cognitive decline than those with normal sensory function.[12,15] Interventions to address these are a potent way to reduce decline and dementia risk.[13] Age-related sensory infirmities, can be insidious in onset and go unrecognized as they mimic the symptoms of neurodegeneration that form the basis of our fears. Get those eyes and ears checked out!

Promote cognitive health:[5,180] Be socially and intellectually involved and engage in lifelong learning. Get adequate sleep and receive treatment for sleep disorders if needed. If hospitalized, discuss available measures to avoid delirium with your care team.[494,495] (See Age-Friendly Health Systems and Geriatric Emergency Departments, mentioned later in this section.)

Carefully evaluate products and services advertised to consumers, such as medications, supplements, and cognitive training. For example, from the World Health Organization and the Institute of Medicine: "Vitamins B and E, polyunsaturated fatty acids and multi-complex supplementation should not be recommended to reduce the risk of cognitive decline and/or dementia."[180] While cognitive stimulation and training can improve older persons' performance on *specific* trained tasks, there are mixed results on the transfer of training effects to new tasks, especially complex everyday activities (such as using a bank's automated teller machine, ATM).[5]

Prevent Worsening after Hospitalization or an Emergency Room (ER) Visit

Consequences of any injury or illness are worse for the elderly with dementia. They are at risk for unexpected deterioration, even after necessary and beneficial contact with any level of hospital-based care.[383,384,483]

Emergency Room (ER) risks:[483,496] The body's ability to compensate for and recover from even minor health problems decreases dramatically with age. Elderly patients discharged from the ER, even after minor injuries or illnesses, are at high risk of functional decline, increased use of health services, reduced health-related quality of life, and death. Within thirty days of an ER discharge, 15–34% of community-dwelling patients over the age of sixty-five experienced an unplanned early return. Within seven days after an ER discharge, 4.5% of older Medicare patients will have a hospital inpatient admission and 0.1–0.5% will die or be admitted to an intensive care unit. Ninety-day mortality for older patients after ER discharge was 10.5%.[483,496]

Risks associated with hospital admission: Hospital admission rates are up to one and a half times higher for elderly patients with dementia when compared with age-matched controls with the same medical diagnoses.[383] "Post-hospital syndrome" refers to functional decline observed in about 35% of geriatric patients after hospital discharge, and the contribution of this phenomenon to short-term return ER visits and repeat hospitalization.[483,497,498]

Nursing homes and "rehab": Elderly patients are frequently discharged from the hospital to a skilled nursing facility for post-acute care. Those whose behavioral problems exceed the facility's capabilities are at high risk of rehospitalization, transfer to another nursing home, or "getting stuck" in long-term care.[384]

Do your research now. Locate an "Age-Friendly Health System" in your area and check it out (http://www.ihi.org /Engage/Initiatives/Age-Friendly-Health-Systems/Pages /default.aspx).[384] "Geriatric Emergency Departments" developed in the last decade offer specialized protocols and expertise. These include post-discharge follow-up tied to early intervention strategies, and specially designed treatment areas to optimize care and transitions of care for older adults.[483] Comprehensive geriatric assessments (CGA) provided by in such units by expert geriatric emergency nurses were associated with decreased inpatient admissions through the emergency department, and decreased costs of inpatient and emergency care.[499]

Identify and Avoid Unreliable Sources of Information

This is only one book, a couple of hundred pages of the best and most up-to-date information that I could find for myself, and then share with you. My conclusions are backed both by more than five hundred verifiable scientific sources and my fifty-plus years of critically evaluating such data. However, when this book is back on your shelf, you are like all of us, stuck in a blizzard of information of widely varying quality and intent. Together, let's review the good and the bad of what we are unavoidably exposed to as we navigate getting older.

Be skeptical. *The most easily triggered red flag should be the realization that somebody is trying to sell you something.* (See also chapter 5.) *Caveat emptor!* The smoothest voice, most familiar face, or most reassuring testimonials are often flawed. "Preliminary" (a.k.a. *unverified*) information is published all the time. In general, try to avoid the shiny object in the newsfeed about AD.

The Limitations of Science

Be cautious about drawing conclusions for *yourself* from the studies discussed here. Much of what we've reviewed derives from comparing large *groups* over time and reporting the percentages in each group who develop the condition under study (*the odds*). No esoteric statistical comparison between populations can translate into the ability to predict *one person's fate*. A simplistic example of a typical between-groups design might compare groups of otherwise similar cognitively normal elders (like cat owners vs. dog owners) for the percentage who develop AD over the length of the study. Applying such "percentage of the group" data to oneself resembles the predicament that arises when someone diagnosed with an early-stage cancer looks up "survival rates" (again, "the odds"). *There is no way for any individual to predict what their personal course will be.*

Even the FDA can get it wrong. (See the treatment section, chapter 5, regarding Aducanumab (Aduhelm®).) Dementia research is high volume, but very low and slow yield. Before the extensively criticized FDA emergency authorization of Aduhelm® in 2021, there had not been a new Alzheimer's drug approved in the preceding eighteen years. All agents previously (and still) on the market are only for treating symptoms. None has yet met the goal of (and the desperate need for) an "effective disease-modifying treatment."

"Initial reports" with encouraging information are continually presented at scientific meetings or offered in press releases from sponsoring institutions, pharmaceutical manufacturers, or device developers. Researchers understandably get excited about early and "suggestive" findings. They want to share their excitement and optimism with the public and their peers (as well as grab credit and acquire funding). Without intentionally misleading, authors and their backers are always eager to maximize the "potential" of their results and minimize any downsides.

Change is slow and incremental, and any source (including this book) may be missing some promising, new information. Find a doctor who keeps up with research and will do so on your behalf.

The media: Nuggets of hope will be picked up by an eager fourth estate and passed on to a desperate public well before they can be verified, peer-reviewed, replicated in a different setting, tested clinically, approved by regulators, and accepted by the Alzheimer's community in general. Medical newsletters, blogs, and other means targeting professionals must attract eyeballs and advertisers to survive.

An audience desperate for good news in the treatment of AD is everywhere. So far, most such "breakthroughs" fail subsequent scrutiny, but not before generating excited stories in print, broadcast, or digital media, and often wildly fluctuating social media speculation. When hopeful bubbles burst, retractions and corrections are often hard to find.

Many commercial news sources gather readers by repackaging preliminary reports from scientific journals or presentations at (often industry-sponsored) meetings to which their audiences may not have access. Key words used in such articles, and particularly their titles, are conspicuous clues to the frequently tenuous and premature nature of these "newsworthy" findings. Examples include: "ASSOCIATION between," "TIED to," "RISK of," "RELATED to," "SUGGESTING a link," "PRELUDE to," "PROMISING," even "NEW." Misleading titles ending in a seemingly breathless question mark are particularly common.

The formula for dubious headlines is well-established: "Persons who (fill in the blank), may be (more/less) likely to develop dementia." Above all, the word *"may"* is number one in what I refer to as "the vernacular of hope and disappointment"—the list of words that authors or reporters of early studies use to try to elevate our interpretation of their findings from a demonstrated association to imply causation.

You'll make yourself crazy looking at every publication (even from reliable sources) that suggests a "link" between AD and something you've already done or is impossible

---

to avoid. While scanning news sources over a two-month period, I came across the following examples, all presented as factors that "may" either promote or inhibit dementia: bilingualism,[500] childhood nightmares,[309] multitasking,[501] gum disease,[502] household chores,[503] a magnesium-rich diet,[504] regular laxative use,[505] stress levels,[506] restless leg syndrome,[507] nose-picking,[508] bone density,[509] and road noise.[312] A current favorite is the online pop-up:

"Scratching THIS Body Part Is a Sign of Alzheimer's."

Such "Over-hyped (Medical) News" is not restricted to Alzheimer's disease and dementia:

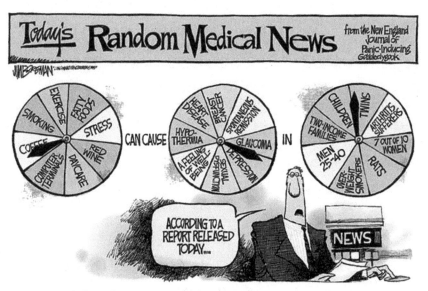

© Jim Borgman – USA TODAY NETWORK

(For a list of the more generally accepted "Potentially Modifiable AD Risk Factors" see chapter 4, table 2.)

Don't read every little blurb and think it's about you and your risks. Don't follow fads. Don't get your advice from advertisements or the Internet. Deception (and outright fraud) are common. Much of the information out there is at best naïve opinion, at worst wishful thinking, paid endorsement, or counterfeit. Sources of information often have impressive names but nothing under the hood. Watch out for "fake news" and even "fake organizations" (see below). Nowhere is it harder for the average person to detect fake news than in fake medical news. Testimonials are useless, not science, and are usually paid for. My real patients were rarely so photogenic, nor so complimentary and concisely articulate. Plant-based products vary in potency with growing-season, weather, soil conditions, plant genetics, storage, additives, and processing. Be skeptical of the "science," "scientists," "scientific publications," and "clinical studies" underlying supplement claims. "Clinical research" that is universally supportive of the product in question, and proudly cited on websites and in advertising materials, is often bogus. Be aware of the existence of literally thousands of so-called "predatory," or "pay-to-publish" pseudo-journals that offer *online-only "publication"* to any writer for a fee, with no peer-review or editing.[510] The phony journal names always sound impressive or closely resemble legitimate scientific publications. Alleged "research" published in such journals often ends up as supportive references in the "published work/scientific research" sections of phony products' websites or ads.

The most (in)famous example may be a paper submitted to, "accepted" by, and "published" online (for a $150 fee) by the International Journal of Advanced Computer Technology. The title was "Get Me Off Your F***ing Mailing List." The text of the "published" ten-page paper (supplemented

---

with a graph and flow chart) consisted entirely of that seven-word phrase repeated over-and-over (https://www.vox.com/2014/11/21/7259207/scientific-paper-scam).

Avoid the Alzheimer's Organization—Do Not Confuse It with the Alzheimer's Association

What follows is my strongly held personal opinion.

It is based on the readily verifiable facts cited below:

My least favorite, and the most dubious example of an unreliable source is a sneaky soundalike, The Alzheimer's Organization (AO); (https://www.alzheimersorganization.org).

It is not the non-profit Alzheimer's Association® (alz.org), which deserves our respect and support, nor is it Alzheimers.gov from the U.S. Department of Health and Human Services. Easily found evidence of what I consider to be their lack of credibility follows:

If you search for "Alzheimer's organizations" on Google, their site shows up in the purchased advertising space halfway down the first page. It is the only website on that page with the subtitle "Information and PRODUCTS [emphasis added] for Alzheimer's disease." It had been one of the more active AD sites on the web, dispensing uncorroborated advice and ending up frequently in my searches. As of July 15, 2022 (and for at least the two preceding years) the address listed on their website for the AO primary office is the same building and suite number as a three-doctor ophthalmology practice offering "premium cataract surgery," whose bona fides I have not investigated. Google Maps and the AO website show that building as immediately adjacent to and apparently on the same campus as a local hospital affiliated with the Cleveland Clinic (an example of the "quality by association" logical fallacy). I make no judgements from the fact that the second-closest medical facility is a pet hospital. Google notwithstanding, AO is not among the sixteen Alzheimer's disease resource-organizations listed by the American Academy of Neurology on their excellent website, www.brainandlife.org.[503]

The "Alzheimer's Organization Mission Statement" reads: "The Alzheimer's Organization was founded by a group of medical professionals affected both personally and professionally by Alzheimer's and dementia. Our goal is to provide information, PRODUCTS [emphasis added], and other resources that will better enable individuals to protect themselves and their loved ones from Alzheimer's and dementia."

No doctors of any type are named on the website. If a "group of medical professionals" (to be fair, they never SAY doctors) won't list their names, degrees, licenses, and specialty certification in front of the public that they are asking for money and confidence (apparently in that order), their offerings do not inspire trust. No scientific references are cited. In my opinion (No References = No Science). They sell vitamins, supplements, and genetic tests for APOE. While "a portion of all proceeds go to support Alzheimer's research," the "portion" is unspecified, as are any specific research recipients. The site comes with the usual supplement disclaimer: "This website does not provide, and should not be used for, medical advice, diagnosis, or treatment. You should consult with your healthcare providers when making decisions regarding your health."

AMEN!

"Propaganda" is Another Word for "Marketing"

What about Prevagen®? Every somewhat sluggish but seemingly happy person in the commercials airing during the evening news is reaching for it. Prevagen® specifically has been thoroughly debunked and its manufacturer successfully sued for millions (see chapter 5). Other "brain booster" products are everywhere and have been subject to similar FDA and legal censures. They lurk in every possible advertising medium among other unsupported claims for "male enhancement," "immune system enrichment," longevity, weight loss, "healthy venous function," "anti-aging" wrinkle creams, and soooo many more.

Beware of testimonials from celebrities and others. Some have even been published without the person's knowledge. (e.g., Denzel Washington and Stephen Hawking were falsely "credited" with promoting Brain-Boosting Pills[511]). Many other public personalities promote products or books for profit. Don't let the fact that such hucksters are often well-known physicians (e.g., Dr. Oz, Dr. Ben Carson) alter your skepticism. There are no cures for aging, avarice, or Alzheimer's disease. If it seems to good to be true . . .

Watch for ID theft and scams. Any of your personal online activity demonstrating an interest in topics related to memory and aging paints a bullseye on your computer's IP address. You might as well change your email address to OldAndVulnerable@ TakeMyMoney.com.

Advanced Directives (Your "Living Will" and "POLST")

If you're old enough to worry about AD, you're old enough to get this aspect of your affairs in order, whether or not you're currently having issues with memory or cognition. Make your wishes known and legally binding. Too many of us put it off. An advanced directive ("living will") conveys the *patient's* end of life wishes. Such personal statements are often best combined with a "POLST" form ("Physician Orders for Life Sustaining Treatment" or, more simply, "Portable Medical Orders").

POLST is a *doctor's order* addressing critical medical decisions that directs and ensures that those wishes are carried out. It is equivalent to in-hospital DNR (do not resuscitate) status, "appropriate for those with a serious illness or frailty near the end-of-life." "Portable" means that the order is valid outside the doctor's office, like a drug prescription, and applies to nursing home and EMS personnel. Though valid nationally, POLST goes by different names in different states (see www.polst.org).

Unfortunately, people sometimes make decisions about their advanced directives based on stigma or fear associated with dementia, or a strong wish not to be dependent on others. They choose to avoid any prolongation of a life with dementia, regardless of its quality and the quality of care they are provided. It is sometimes suggested that if people lack confidence that they will be able to exert some control over their health care at the end of life, they may prefer to consider suicide or some form of assisted dying as a way of taking more direct, personal control at an earlier stage in the illness.[486] A best practice would be early discussions with family and other trusted advisors, culminating in unambiguous powers of attorney and advance directives that fully account for one's feelings on issues like quality of life and dignity.

I strongly recommend reviewing the writings of Norman L. Cantor, a distinguished professor of law and bioethics. I have used (and credited) his thoughts and words to formulate my own advance directive, should I reach (in his words) "the point of intolerable cognitive decline triggering medical nonintervention."[512] I've cared for thousands of elderly patients with cognitive decline and with their families at the bedside. My personal standard for "pulling the plug" on myself (or in Cantor's words, expressing the wish that "life-preserving medical treatment be withheld or withdrawn") has rarely resembled what I have so often heard from my dementia patients' family members and decision-makers. Their thoughts on what their *own* wishes might be in similar circumstances were often expressed (in a bedside whisper) as: "If I ever get this way, just shoot me!" My choice to shun a well-meaning bullet in favor of a thoughtful advance directive comes from attending and interacting over the decades with so many "pleasantly demented" older patients of mine. Such "shoot me" statements, seemed to me to be less in response to their loved-one's objective situation, than they were to the stresses of caregiving, and the anxiety of imagining themselves in such a state. Many of those demented patients of mine had a much better quality of life than nursing-home patients I cared for without dementia, for whom no one was considering euthanasia. *Quality of life from the patient's perspective is my recommended decision framework.* Look at their face and body language when they are having "a good day."

As is appropriate to the topic, Cantor's strong and articulate views are admittedly personal. "Some people will confront Alzheimer's with a measure of resignation, a determination to struggle against the progressive debilitation and to extract whatever comforts and benefits they can from their remaining existence. They are entitled to pursue that resolute path. For other people, like myself, protracted maintenance during progressive cognitive dysfunction and helplessness is an intolerably degrading prospect."[512]

His 1990 article, "My Annotated Living Will"[513] forms the basis of my own advance medical directive. It is the only such document I have seen that defines the demented state in terms of the individual's experienced quality of life (as opposed to idiosyncratic external interpretations of what a loving and well-meaning person thinks it would be like to "live that way"). Cantor clearly articulates the thoughts that I want included in decision-making on my behalf. He plainly defines concepts and obligations like: medical intervention is to be guided by *"my best interests;"* and recognizes "pleasantly demented" as OK (see also, *Newsweek*, September 2, 2008[514]). "Capacity for sentient existence" is primary, while a "demeaning or degrading mental state," "physical indignity," and "helplessness" are "intolerable."[513] Your mileage may vary, but the paper deserves a thoughtful look from anyone crafting their advanced directive/health care power of attorney.

Thanks to the generosity of the publisher, The American Society of Law, Medicine, and Ethics, any reader may request a free scanned copy of Cantor's "annotated living will" by sending an email to publications@aslme.org (The article is identified as: Cantor, N. L. (1990). "My Annotated Living Will." Law Med Health Care 18(1-2): 114-122. doi: 10.1111/j.1748-720x.1990.tb01139.x. PMID: 2374443).

Getting on with Life After a Diagnosis

Adopt systems to replace reliance on short-term memory. There are books for this. Form useful habits. Leave a to-do list for your aging self. Always keep those notepads, wayward keys, and eyeglasses in their own space. Start early.

Maximally utilize your biological clock. The distinctions between people who are "early birds" versus those who are "night owls" have been well studied. Some times of day (driven by your unique circadian rhythms and/or environment) will be consistently more productive than others. Recognize and utilize your most functional periods to complete tasks and make plans with optimal clarity.[515]

Acquire a pet, one with care requirements that match your time and capabilities. An animal companion provides a comforting relationship that transcends language, memory, and cognition. You can never have too much love in your life. An advanced dementia patient and dog lover I knew gained obvious pleasure and comfort from interacting with a mechanical canine.

Driving: AARP has advice and information for patients and families. Online and classroom courses can confirm and improve your safety behind the wheel. Rehabilitation centers can provide objective physician-guided assessments that mesh with legal requirements.

Contribute to research if you can, personally and financially.

Connect! You are not alone. Nearly everyone our age will be confronted with similar concerns for themselves or a loved one. We all have same-age friends. We can provide a support group for ourselves, helping each other in person or expand mutually beneficial connections through an online community. There is a lot of help out there: AARP, alz.org, community resources, specialized centers, and local and national support groups. (See Appendix II – Resources.)

Plan ahead with family and others for the practical aspects and details of decline. A useful source discussed in chapter 4 is: *The Complete Bedside Companion: A No-Nonsense Advice On Caring for the Seriously Ill* by Rodger McFarlane and Philip Basche.[380]

Take stock of family resources to better predict the need for outside help. Who is nearby? How might distant relatives share responsibility?

Use technology to expand safety and prolong independent living with medical or behavioral monitoring from a distance. Think voice assistants and other assistive technology.

Caring for Those with Dementia (see also chapter 4)

Day-to-Day

Remember that those with dementia, especially in the earlier stages, retain the capacity to make many decisions, especially when supported in doing so. How things are done, ensuring that people with dementia feel valued as individuals, will often be far more important than the exact format of the service provided.

One cannot underestimate the importance of support for caretakers, family members, and involved friends. Their well-being is critical for optimal care and integral to maintaining relationships which are central and centering for many people with dementia.

The 'little things' of care are particularly important in enhancing autonomy and well-being. The humanity with which assistance for everyday living is offered, especially help with eating and intimate care, is crucial to retaining self-esteem and dignity. Similarly significant are the manner and tone in which a person is addressed; the care taken to ensure that they participate as much as they can, or wish to, in any decision about their day-to-day life; the trouble taken about appropriate and attractive food and environments; and access to meaningful activity."[486]

Anticipate progression and prevent the consequences: e.g., depression (discuss treatment, optimize behavioral interventions, and get firearms out of the house); accidents in the home (kitchen fires, fall prevention); outside the home (driving, getting lost, assaults); fraud and worse: risk of ID theft, robbery, assault.

Ethical Considerations[486]

Restraint: The course of dementia (with its loss of cognitive capacity and independence, and associated changes in mood) is both highly distressing to the patient and frustrating for caregivers. The potential for frequent conflicts creates ethical as well as practical difficulties. Ethical issues include methods used to control or prevent a person's spontaneous behaviors. Restraint can include using or threatening force to overcome a person's resistance, or restricting their movements, whether or not they resist. Techniques include physically holding a person, using straps or belts to keep them in a chair, locking doors, and using drugs to calm and control. In some circumstances, a person with dementia may understand why a particular restriction is being suggested for their own safety and may consent to its use. In other cases, however, they may not be able to consent, or restraint may be used to control behavior that others find difficult or alarming. In such cases, restraint may be experienced as highly demeaning and distressing. Yet, at times, those caring for a person with dementia may see no alternative. For people who lack capacity to consent, regulations may limit the use of restraint to circumstances where it is "proportionate" to the likelihood of the person suffering harm.

    Conflicting needs: The requirements of the person with dementia will sometimes conflict with the desires of others who also deserve consideration. A spouse is the primary example.

    Research ethics and poorly validated "innovative practice": The frustrating lack of disease-modifying treatments for Alzheimer's has led to what some argue are premature *innovative practices*, lacking evidence from the usual confirmatory studies traditionally conducted in very large health systems. Such nonvalidated approaches raise several ethical questions: how to responsibly apply such practice to individual patients, the way such "innovations" are communicated or promoted by the scientific and lay press, and the appropriateness of making such practices widely available before more definitive testing.[467,468]

Palliative Care: How Would You Like to be Treated?

Evidence suggests that individuals with dementia are less likely to receive end-of-life care comparable to that provided to those without dementia. Dementia patients are less commonly referred to palliative care specialists, receive palliative medication, or have attention paid to their spiritual needs.[486] Failure to adopt a palliative or holistic supportive approach can occur because those with advanced dementia may not be perceived as suffering from a "terminal illness." Because of the often-uncertain time course of a dementia prognosis, criteria for hospice care are not commonly met.

Be aware of the following unsettling statistics. Consider them when planning for later stages of care.[368,373]

(1) A study comparing symptoms experienced in the last year of life by dementia and cancer patients showed that the symptom burden was comparable between the two groups.

(2) Medical and nursing home staff consistently overestimate prognosis in advanced dementia. Upon nursing home admission, only 1% of new residents were perceived to have a life expectancy of less than six months, yet 71% died within that period.

(3) "Despite the high mortality in advanced dementia, particularly for those who are admitted to acute-care hospitals, people with dementia received as many painful investigations and procedures and were more likely to be physically restrained compared with patients who are cognitively intact."[368]

Important Details and Administrative Housekeeping

While I have attempted to make this manuscript as comprehensive as possible, there are far better resources than I for such topics. Personal attorneys, other trusted advisors, and the AARP are probably among the most reliable. (See Appendix II—Resources.)

Legal Issues

These include the following: competency, capacity, danger to self or others, wills, trusts, medical and financial powers of attorney, and advance directives.

"Competency" is a *legal* determination of one's ability to manage some or all of their affairs. "Competency" is determined by a judge.

"Capacity" is a *medical* determination. Can a patient, at a particular moment, consent to or refuse proposed care? Capacity requires the abilities to understand the nature of one's illness; the risks, benefits, and alternatives of a proposed intervention; and to make a reasoned decision to accept or reject care. For example, a patient out of touch with reality from acute psychosis may lack capacity. Specifics may vary in different states or countries.[516] One way to hopefully reduce problems inherent in borderline capacity is having an early agreement on joint decision-making with trusted family members, bridging the gap to the time when formal proxy decision-making, like powers of attorney, becomes necessary.[486]

Finances: Issues include day-to-day bill paying, funerals, paying down assets to qualify for Medicaid and nursing home care, community services, elder lawyers, inheritance, property, wills, and trusts. Long-term care insurance is not an affordable or appropriate option for everyone, but everyone should investigate it and make a judgement for themselves. Policies can include payments for in-home care.

Security: Write down where important items and papers can be found for yourself and for family and tell family and trusted counselors where the list is. Safeguard passwords, bank and brokerage accounts, keys, credit cards, policies, heirlooms, wills, and car titles. Protect against scammers and identity theft.

What if you have no one? With financial resources: consider guardianship by an elder-law firm. Don't leave it to the state; do it while you have your faculties. In the absence of resources: legal aid, petitions for guardianship, Medicaid, Adult Protective Services, the local Area Agency on Aging, social services.

Activism

IF YOU REMEMBER ANYTHING, REMEMBER THE SIXTIES: AGEISM IS A CIVIL RIGHTS ISSUE.

Take Control

Don't let the bastards get you down. Leave your mark. Say your piece. It helps. Nothing improves the fluency of my speech more than annoyance. Don't fall into the trap of playing the nice old geezer: smiling politely at "OK, boomer," or responding "It's good to be seen." Bullshit! Call out that ageist crap! To quote author and investment advisor @brianportnoy (Twitter, Apr 22, 2019): "Free advice: When someone says "It's good to see you," do not reply, "It's good to be seen." You'll sound like a d*ck."

I'm not a violent person; my last physical confrontation was in sixth grade. Yet, every time the sweet gray-haired lady behind the counter at the convenience store calls me "young fella" I visualize myself leaping over the lottery machine to waterboard her with a Piña Colada Slurpee.

Look at the bright side: even if mentation declines, longstanding dreams may still come true. I have often said, not totally in jest, that if I ever received a terminal diagnosis, I would do two things that would give me pleasure: (1) take up smoking again (last pack of Luckies, 1969; still miss one after a good meal) and (2) start saying out loud all the things that I was only thinking, but always really ached to say. I used to warn Security at my last hospital to lock the doors if they ever saw me coming smoking a cigarette. No one there would want to hear what I had to say.

A note to my health-care "team": Count me among the 60% of patients who find being addressed as "Honey," "Sweetheart," "Dear," etc. to be "disrespectful, patronizing and overly familiar." [517]

Have some fun with it. No stranger knows what your "normal aging" should look like. Create your own expectations. Be "eccentric." Don't apologize. They can't blame the old fella they think has dementia. Call them out for ageism. Embrace the freedom of not remembering.

Fight Back: Don't get mad, get even: leave the toilet seat up, belch, use your cane, go ahead and fart, forget to pay, let the door close in their faces: "Oops, sorry young fella."

Combine Forces: Band together at the senior center, day care, VA, VFW, assisted living, or nursing home to fight for equal rights. Utilize the "wisdom of the crowd," and potentially, the Americans with Disabilities Act.

WORK on OUR problems: The path to the dementia pigeonhole is a lot longer than those who define us by our looks, our clothes, our driving, our choices in music, and our senior discounts, think it is. Treat me like the person with the bad leg getting out of the car in the handicapped spot. I may need help opening the door, but it doesn't mean I can't find it. Be kind. Be a Scout, but don't be prejudiced or make assumptions about me based on age, some hearing loss, and the occasional conversational *non sequitur*.

Discrimination against the "memory-challenged elderly" should energize a fight for our rights, as others with disabilities continue to do. The expression "senior moment" is an ageist attribution. Increasing use of the phrase suggests that negative stereotypes of older adults remain socially acceptable.[518] My bad!: I recognize that I have used "senior moment" ten times in this book, mostly when discussing a journal reference that used the phrase, and well before I was moved to author this paragraph. In calling out friends, relatives, and strangers for their "ageist attribution," I mean no more disrespect than do those who use the expression in referring to me and my contemporaries. "Sorry, young fella."

People should cut us the same sort of slack in conversation that they do for those other seniors in parking lots. Communication during my four-decade emergency medicine career was likely around 80% talk and 20% writing. Presenting my findings and recommendations coherently, and in a manner tailored to the patient and family in front of me, is what got me over the finish line in persuading tens of thousands of them to follow any of my advice, from "Good news, it's just a cold, no prescription needed," to "While indigestion is still a possibility, sir, your age, sky-high blood pressure, and abnormal electrocardiogram suggest you should stay in the hospital to further evaluate and treat your heart attack." It is easy for me to imagine how my progressive word-finding difficulties would likely have qualified as a serious challenge at work. Credible, concise, and effective verbal communication is fundamental to medicine and many other occupations and is hard to achieve when one is visibly and haltingly searching for the right words. <u>Consider my nightmare at 3 a.m. example: "Nurse, give Mr. _____ an amp of that heart-starty stuff, STAT!"</u>

Unfortunately, age often takes our voices when we need them the most. While we can, we should organize families, legislators, businesses, and the health-care industry to pick up the slack and support official "Handicapped" status for memory-impaired elders.

Conclusion: There Is Hope

Progression to AD is *not* Inevitable

A survey of seventy thousand people from 155 countries found that a quarter believed that there is nothing that can ever be done to prevent dementia.[519] Not true! The lifetime risk of dementia is 37% for women and 24% for men.[150] Even "at 100 years or older, high levels of cognitive performance can be maintained for several years, even when individuals are exposed to risk factors associated with cognitive decline."[520,521] "The pessimism felt by those who assume that dementia is an inevitable consequence of ageing, or that a positive family history of dementia indicates that they will follow the same course, is misplaced."[522] For example, managing cardiovascular risks could prevent up to a third of all dementias.[523] (See risk factor modification, chapter 5.)

"They're Working Hard on This"

> If you are reading (or writing) a book about memory and dementia, "every slip seems like a fall." We all have "moments" at any age. Much is still in your hands. Keep going! Even if lifestyle modification doesn't work on memory, it can't hurt to be healthier.

The massive numbers of scientists attacking this problem worldwide have uncovered, in just the last few years, a plethora of new information. As just one example, the published proceedings of the 14th Clinical Trials on Alzheimer's Disease Symposium contained 168 pages of posters, symposia, conferences, and oral communication abstracts, with multiple abstracts per page.[524,525] Real progress *will* follow.

Keep reading and educating yourself and your doctors. New information will continue coming out at an increased rate as more investigators and individuals get touched by AD and live longer.

"Ultimately, there will be a future in which specific anti-Alzheimer's therapy will be combined with lifestyle interventions targeting general brain health to jointly combat the disease."[55]

Clinical trials may be considered (with good risk/benefit discussion) at major medical centers. Include family and respected advisors in the decision.

Here's some hopeful news: "The prevalence of dementia in the United States declined significantly between 2000 and 2016.

A substantial increase in the overall level of education was associ-ated with the largest decline in dementia prevalence,[526] but "the full set of social, behavioral, and medical factors contributing to the decline is still uncertain."[527] The prevalence of dementia is declining in Europe as well, and is also likely multifactorial.[528] Incidence in the western world may have decreased as a result of better vascular care and improved overall health.[55,424]

This book is for you, so use the information provided. When your adult kids start making fun of your senior moments, share the statistics with them. Point them towards known preventive measures that will contribute to *their* overall health and longevity. Seek out the best doctors. Get your wellness shit together. Donate to Alzheimer's research. Plan, with your family, for the future.

If you are "of an age" reading this, and have no symptoms, congratulations! Just continue doing what you're doing—it seems to be working! For now, put down the book and go be with your grandkids.

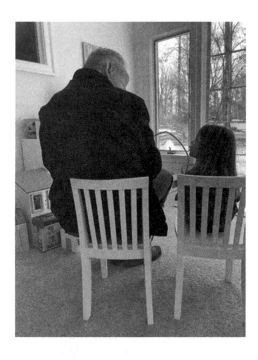

APPENDIX I: GLOSSARY

ACRONYMS, ABBREVIATIONS, and DEFINITIONS

ACR—Annual Conversion Rate
Rate of progression from one diagnosis to the next; most severe in the sequence from the pre-symptomatic stage of Alzheimer's disease to dementia.

AD—Alzheimer's Disease (see chapter 4)
The term reserved for cases where neuropathologic or bio-marker evidence of the disease is present.

ADLs—Activities of daily living, the "functional" impairments that come with progressive cognitive loss. They are activities related to personal care, and include bathing or showering, dressing, getting in and out of a bed or chair, walking, using the toilet, and eating. Failure to perform ADLs (in the absence of other causes) defines dementia.

Alzheimer's Clinical Syndrome
The recommended terminology for a clinically diagnosed memory loss without biomarker confirmation of AD. Occurring in both mildly impaired and demented individuals, this is what has historically been labeled "possible or probable AD."

ADAS-Cog—Alzheimer's Disease Assessment Scale-Cognitive Subscale
An early (1980s) and frequently modified neuropsychological measure used in AD research trials, it measures several cognitive domains, including memory, language and praxis with both subject-completed tests and observer-based assessments.

ADRD—Alzheimer's disease and related dementias

AHRQ—Agency for Healthcare Research and Quality

aMCI—Amnestic mild cognitive impairment (see chapter 3)

Anomia
A form of aphasia in which the patient is unable to recall the names of everyday objects.

Aphasia
Trouble speaking or understanding other people speaking due to damage or disruptions in parts of the brain that control spoken language.

APOE
A gene with subtypes that produces proteins implicated in both Alzheimer's disease and cardiovascular disease (APOE4)

ARML—Age-Related Memory Loss

ARCD—Age-Related Cognitive Decline
Deterioration in cognitive performance that can be a normal part of aging. It is also sometimes referred to as cognitive aging.

ATN—**A**myloid, Pathologic **T**au, and **N**eurodegeneration/ neuronal injury
A biomarker classification system. Each of these three measurable pathologic processes of AD are labelled as either normal ("1") or abnormal ("2"). The possibilities of three markers and two states (normal/abnormal) for each establishes eight possible biomarker profiles for any individual (e.g. A1T2(N)2, A1T1(N)2, etc.). The profiles define three patient *biomarker categories*: (1) normal AD biomarkers, (2) on the Alzheimer's

continuum; and (3) non-Alzheimer's pathologic change (i.e., suspected non-Alzheimer's pathophysiology or SNAP).

BDNF—Brain-Derived Neurotrophic Factor
A genetically regulated brain protein important for neuronal survival and growth. It serves as a neurotransmitter modulator and participates in neuronal plasticity—essential for learning and memory.

CATD—Clinical Alzheimer's-Type Dementia
"Clinical Alzheimer's-type" acknowledges the presence of dementia severe enough to limit independent functioning, but without biomarker evidence of AD-related brain changes (biomarker testing negative or not performed). This label is used infrequently and may accompany one of the less common causes, or a "mixed" number of causes of dementia (see chapter 4).

CDR—Clinical Dementia Rating
Ratings are assigned on a 0–5 point scale, from 0 = absent to 5 = terminal, and can be used to group together patients with the same severity of dementia for study.

Cognition
The term *cognition* covers many mental processes, including decision-making, memory, attention, perception, thinking, understanding, learning, language use, and problem-solving.

Cognitive Decline/Cognitive Impairment
"Cognitive decline, which is characterized by deterioration in processing speed, attention, reasoning, spatial perception and memory, is considered a normal part of aging."[329]

CI—Confidence Interval
Statistics: a range of values so defined that there is a specified probability (often 95%) that the value of a parameter of interest lies within the described range.

Cognitive Domains[206,529]
Cognition is typically subdivided into tiered domains of function. These domains are hierarchical. Basic sensory and perceptual processes are on the bottom, with the top domains exerting executive functions and cognitive control over the use of more basic processes. Cognitive domains include complex attention, executive function, learning and memory, language, perceptual-motor control, and social cognition.

Cognitive Reserve
An individual's unique capacity to maintain normal cognitive function in the presence of brain disease or injury.

Comorbidity
The simultaneous presence of two or more diseases or medical conditions in a patient.

"Cover Boy"
Answer to chapter 1 quiz: Alfred E. Neuman, *MAD* magazine, "What, Me Worry?"

COX-2—Cyclooxygenase-2
Is the enzyme responsible for causing inflammation. Nonsteroidal anti-inflammatory drugs inhibit COX-2.

DASH—Dietary Approaches to Stop Hypertension

Delirium
Delirium is a clinical syndrome that usually develops in the elderly. Characterized by an alteration of attention, consciousness, and cognition, delirium develops rapidly and *fluctuates* during the day. By definition, delirium is caused by an underlying medical condition and is not better explained by a neurocognitive disorder.

Differential Diagnosis
A medical differential diagnosis is both a (1) *list* of conditions that share the same symptoms and (2) the name of the *process* (often tests) by which conditions on the list are excluded to get to the most accurate diagnosis. For example, a simple upper respiratory infection ("common cold") will often have an associated cough, as will a more serious lung infection (pneumonia). Both conditions (and some others) are in the differential diagnosis, the list of conditions, that can cause cough. Two tests common in the process of differentiating the causes of a cough would be taking a temperature and obtaining a chest X-ray. Both should be normal with a cold and are more likely to be abnormal with pneumonia.

Disinhibition
Literally, the loss or reduction of an inhibition, resulting in poorly controlled or poorly restrained emotions or actions. manifested in disregard of social conventions, impulsivity, and poor risk assessment.

ECOG Scale—Eastern Cooperative Oncology Group (ECOG) Performance Status
Scale used to describe a patient's level of functioning in terms of their ability to care for themself, daily activity, and physical ability levels. Ranges from 0 (fully active, no performance

restrictions) to 4 (completely disabled; cannot carry out any self-care; totally confined to bed or chair).

EPC—Evidence-Based Practice Center

Executive Functions

The higher-level cognitive skills one uses to control and coordinate their other cognitive abilities and behaviors. Multiple lists exist. Most include high-order cognitive abilities such as working memory, inhibitory control, cognitive flexibility, planning, reasoning, and problem solving.

"Functional" Abilities

Refers to the ability to perform activities of daily living (ADLs).

"Functional" Illness

Refers to an illness without an identified physical cause, commonly used with psychiatric and neurological disorders.

Genotype

A scoring (description) of an organism's complete hereditary information, even if not expressed.

GDS—Global Deterioration Scale[177]

Describes seven stages of the typical witnessed *clinical* course of AD (ranging from the absence of any subjective or objective abnormalities (GDS 1) to the loss of speech and ambulation (GDS 7).

Heritable (and Heritability)

Tendencies readily passed on from parents to children, but without a particular genetic mechanism or obvious familial pattern (not dominant or recessive). LOAD heritability of late-onset AD accounts for the two-to-threefold increased risk of developing AD in first-degree relatives (siblings, children) of AD patients.

IADL—Instrumental Activity of Daily Living[206]
Light housework, preparing meals, taking medications, shopping for groceries and clothes, using the telephone, managing money and paying bills.

IOM—The Institute of Medicine
The National Academy of Medicine was known as the Institute of Medicine (IOM) until 2015

Lethologica—The Tip-Of-The-Tongue Phenomenon

MAT—Memory Alteration Test
For the purpose of detecting amnestic MCI and early AD in population with low educational level.[530]

MAC-Q—The Memory Assessment Clinic-Q
A six-item scale measuring age-related memory decline. Items are framed to assess change relative to the respondent's own baseline at age twenty.

MCI—Mild Cognitive Impairment (see chapter 3)

Metanalysis or Meta-analysis
The statistical process of analyzing and combining results from several similar studies. By generating an average result, a meta-analysis adds value because it can produce a more precise estimate of the effect of a treatment than considering each study individually.

Metacognition
The awareness and understanding of one's own thought processes. Cognitive decline can occur with or without metacognition.

"Moderate to severe" AD

This phrase refers to clinical stages 5 and 6 in the research definition of AD from the 2018 NIAA-AA International Working Group (IWG). Moderate dementia refers to "extensive functional impact on daily life," no longer independent and requiring frequent assistance with daily life activities. With severe dementia there is "complete dependency" with impairment in basic activities, including simple self-care.[49]

Neurobehavioral Symptoms

Symptoms attributable to mood or behavioral disorders; for example, anxiety, depression, and apathy

Neuropsychiatric (a.k.a. Neuropsychological) Testing

Refers to comprehensive testing of multiple cognitive domains performed and interpreted by a specialist. Tests consist variably of questions and answers, paper and pencil tasks, and structured and unstructured interviews, neuropsychological testing evaluates language usage and comprehension, attention/concentration, processing speed, learning and memory, reasoning, visuospatial and motor skills, mood, personality, general intellect, and executive functions.

NIA—National Institute on Aging

NIA-AA—National Institute on Aging and the Alzheimer's Association
A collaborative International Working Group (IWG) of these two organizations formalized both the biological[49] and clinical[226] definitions of Alzheimer's disease.

NIH—National Institutes of Health

NMDA—N-methyl-D-aspartate
Mediator of excitatory neurotransmission in the central nervous system (CNS) with key roles in learning, and memory.

Phenotype
Phenotype refers to an individual's observable traits, such as height, eye color, and blood type. A person's phenotype is determined by the interaction of both their genomic makeup (genotype) and environmental factors.

Praxis
The ability to carry out skilled purposeful movements and gestures when asked. The opposite, "apraxia," is the inability to do so, despite having the desire, understanding, and the physical ability.

"Preclinical" vs. "Prodromal" AD
Preclinical (asymptomatic) AD can be defined as the stage when biomarker changes are present, but clinical symptoms have not yet developed, whereas prodromal AD is usually defined as the earliest stage when cognitive symptoms are present, but the requirements for a dementia diagnosis have not yet been met.

PubMed—National Library of Medicine database of published scientific papers.

RCT—Randomized Controlled Trial
An experimental design that randomly assigns participants into either an experimental group or a control group. The only expected difference between the groups is the outcome variable being studied.

RR—Relative Risk
Compares the risk of a health event (disease, injury, risk factor, or death) within one group with the risk among another group (e.g., women are 100% more likely to give birth than men).

SBP—Systolic Blood Pressure

SCI (Subjective Cognitive Impairment) and SCC (Subjective Cognitive Complaints) —Earlier Labels for SCD (subjective cognitive decline) (See chapter 2)
These terms have been used interchangeably, mainly to describe the population of "worried well." SCI "refers to people who are concerned that they may have dementia, but are neurologically normal relative to others in their demographic upon examination and testing."[95]

SCD—Subjective Cognitive Decline (see chapter 2)

SD—Standard Deviation
The standard deviation measures how spread out data is. It is a measure of how far each observed value is from the mean (average). In any "normal" distribution, about 95% of values will be within two standard deviations of the mean.

Shared Decision-Making
Shared decision-making (SDM) has been defined as "an approach where clinicians and patients share the best available evidence when faced with the task of making decisions, and where patients are supported to consider options to achieve informed preferences."[531]

Sensitivity/Specificity
"Sensitivity" refers to a test's ability to identify a positive result when administered to an individual with a disease. A "highly

sensitive" test means that there are few false negative results, and thus fewer cases of disease are missed.

The "specificity" of a test is its ability to designate as negative an individual who does not have a disease, thus limiting false positives.

Systematic Reviews

Authors of "systematic reviews" gather all relevant studies conducted on a specific clinical question. Then, they evaluate that body of knowledge and combine their findings, using pre-defined, rigorous, and clearly documented methods. If they have found enough high-quality studies, systematic reviews can form the basis for clinical recommendations.

SSRI—Selective Serotonin Reuptake Inhibitors, the most commonly prescribed antidepressants.

USPSTF—U. S. Preventive Services Task Force
"Created in 1984, the U. S. Preventive Services Task Force is an independent volunteer panel of national experts in prevention and evidence-based medicine. The Task Force works to improve the health of people nationwide by making evidence-based recommendations about clinical preventive services such as screenings, counseling services, and preventive medications." (www.uspreventiveservicestaskforce.org.)

Visuospatial Skills

Visuospatial abilities represent a person's capacity to identify visual and spatial relationships among objects. A good example is parking a car.

WHO—World Health Organization

"Worried Complainers"

These are persons whose complaints impact their activities of daily living, and are also noticed by an informant. They have the highest risk of progression to MCI or AD among those with subjective concerns (SCC, SCD, SCI). (Chapter 2.)

"Worried Well"

SCI is a term that describes the population of "worried well." These are people who are concerned that they may have dementia, but upon examination and testing are neurologically normal relative to others in their demographic.[95]

APPENDIX II: RESOURCES

SELECTION OF RESOURCES

An assuredly incomplete list, these are personal opinions generated during the more than three-year process of researching and writing this book. These are not blanket endorsements. They proved helpful in my work, and in my experience have been solid, consistently reliable sources of information on the topics presented.

Helpful Organizations

AARP (www.aarp.org). Always informative and eminently practical, I read their periodicals regularly and usually learn something of value. I find the group to be an excellent source of accurate health information for the general public and frequently recommend AARP as a source to friends and family. Here's just one example: "Don't Just Google Your Symptoms. How to Find Credible Health Info Online" (published in the *AARP Bulletin*, May 2023, pp. 16, 18, 19.)

Full Disclosure: I was compensated at what I assume was AARP's usual rate for the one article that I published in the *AARP Bulletin* in 2021,[496] the only writing for which I had ever been paid. The truly remarkable thoroughness with which their fact-checking staff vetted my every statement and reference in that brief piece forms the strongest basis for my recommendation. In my over fifty years of being published in medical textbooks, basic science and medical journals, and medical newsmagazines, no publication or editor has ever come close to (appropriately) scrutinizing my sources and conclusions so thoroughly.

The Alzheimer's Association (www.alz.org) "Formed in 1980, the Alzheimer's Association is the leading voluntary health organization in Alzheimer's care, support and research."

The American Academy of Neurology maintains a valuable *Brain & Life* website (www.brainandlife.org) and offers a free bimonthly print magazine by the same name. The website includes a searchable database with disorder-specific information about many common brain conditions, including the dementias.

Alzheimer's Disease International (www.alzint.org) partners with the World Health Organization and others along with 120 countries, and publishes a yearly *World Alzheimer's Report.*

The National Institute on Aging (NIA), one of the National Institutes of Health, is the lead federal agency for research on aging, Alzheimer's disease, and related dementias (www.nia.nih.gov). NIA offers excellent free publications specifically directed at our needs. Of particular relevance are: *"What Are Clinical Trials and Studies?"* https://www.nia.nih.gov/health/what-are-clinical-trials-and-studies.

The World Health Organization *(www.who.int)* issues periodic reports on dementia. WHO's "Comprehensive Global Action Plan for the Public Health Response to Dementia" identifies priority action areas, sets targets for countries to achieve, and provides governments with a framework to develop their own national dementia plans.[532] WHO reports accessed for this work include:[163,180,181,519,533]

The Washington State Dementia Action Collaborative (https://tinyurl.com/ytbk5p9w) publishes the *Dementia Road Map: A Guide for Family and Care Partners*. It is comprehensive, up to date, readable, free, and available from the Washington State Department of Social and Health Services at: https://www.dshs.wa.gov/sites/default/files/ALTSA/stakeholders/documents/AD/Dementia%20Road%20Map%20-%20A%20Guide%20for%20Family%20and%20Care%20Partners.pdf.

A Place for Mom (www.aplaceformom.com)
CAUTION: This is (very openly) a for-profit senior care referral service advertised as "free to families." While researching the book, I signed up for their email newsletter. I have no opinion of or experience with the referral services they offer, but their informative newsletter has been an excellent source of readable and practical information on multiple facets of aging, without surprise sales pitches or electronic intrusions.

Scientific References: Obtaining Your Own Copies

Online:

The vast majority of my primary information sources are in scientific journals and written by academic researchers. Written in the language they use to communicate with their peers on topics familiar to both the writer and the reader, these works were never oriented towards the general public. *However, if you wish to acquire any of my original source material, you can!*

Many of the hundreds of references I reviewed that are identified by superscript numbers throughout the text, and fully identified in the section at the end of the book, are readily available for free. Many readers are unaware that any internet access comes with the equivalent of a free (taxpayer-funded) library card providing online privileges at the National Institutes of Health's National Library of Medicine. At their website (pubmed.gov), anyone can readily access the author(s) summary of the paper (known as the "Abstract"), and other valuable information in real time and without registering or fees.

Free full-text copies are often available for download by clicking through from the same site. They are archived in "PubMed Central (PMC)," a repository of articles maintained by the National Institutes of Health (NIH) and other organizations that fund scientific research. Such organizations often require authors they support to upload a copy of their accepted manuscripts to PMC. A great many publications cited in this book fall into this category.

Online access to the National Library of Medicine (pubmed. gov) is free and easy. Instructions for use can be accessed at: https://www.nlm.nih.gov/services/faqimages/locatorplus/Access_Full_Text_at_NLM.doc. Enter enough information to identify the paper you are seeking. Usually, the first author's name and initials, the year, and a unique portion of the title are more than adequate.

From "Brick and Mortar" Libraries:

The reference librarian at your local public library (the big building with the shelves full of actual printed paper books) can often help. Systems and resources will vary by locality. Check their website and/or contact a reference librarian.

Local library memberships often include free electronic access to larger regional and statewide libraries. These larger libraries often subscribe to online databases containing articles you seek. Additionally, many colleges and universities offer some level of online or in-person library privileges to alumnae. Check with your alumnae association.

Interlibrary loan (ILL) from your local library can often acquire electronic versions or photocopies of harder-to-access works for you. There may be a charge, particularly if photo-copying or mailing is required.

Books and Reports Mentioned in the Text

Medical textbook: Budson, A. and P. Solomon. *Memory Loss, Alzheimer's Disease and Dementia*. Philadelphia: Elsevier, 2002. This is the most recent medical textbook on Alzheimer's dis-ease. While intended for the academically inclined and health-care providers (and I have not read the whole thing), it seems to be clearly written, up-to-date, comprehensive, aimed at a more general audience, and offering considerable practical advice.

Caregiving in general: McFarlane, R. and P. Bashe. *The Complete Bedside Companion: No-Nonsense Advice on Caring for the Seriously Ill*. New York: Simon & Schuster, 1998. (Discussed in chapter 4; several used copies available for less than seven dol-lars on Amazon.)

The National Academies Press (NAP) exists to publish (dig-itally and for free) the hundreds of reports issued yearly by the National Academies of Sciences, Engineering, and Medicine (www.nationalacademies.org). These prestigious, private, non-profit institutions offer expert review, analysis and advice on national and international challenges, including those about which this book was written. NAP reports cited in this work include references:[5,160,161,165,183,191,335,375,377,384,534,535]

Local and Regional Resources

State and local health departments
Social services (hospital, community-based, faith-based)
Area Agencies on Aging
Senior community centers

Public library
Volunteer and charity organizations

Unreliable Resources

See chapter 5, "To Be Avoided," and chapter 6.

From chapter 6, but worth repeating: "Avoid the Alzheimer's Organization, and do not confuse it with the Alzheimer's Association."

REFERENCES

1. Jahn H. "Memory loss in Alzheimer's disease." *Dialogues Clin Neurosci.* Dec 2013; 15(4):445-54.

2. Budson AE, Solomon PR. "Appendix C: Memory Dysfunction in Alzheimer's Disease and Other Causes of Mild Cognitive Impairment and Dementia." *Memory Loss, Alzheimer's Disease and Dementia.* 3 ed. Elsevier; 2022:e12-e17.

3. Walinga J, Stranger C. Chapter 9.1 9.1 "Memories as Types and Stages." *Introduction to Psychology - 1st Canadian Edition, 2021.* https://opentextbcca/introductiontopsychology/chapter/8-1-memories-as-types-and-stages/. Accessed June 20, 2021.

4. Meilleur C. "8 Types of Memory… to Remember!" KnowledgeOne, Nov. 9, 2018: https://knowledgeone.ca/8-types-of-memory-to-remember/. Accessed June 23, 2021.

5. *IOM (Institute of Medicine). Cognitive aging: Progress in understanding and opportunities for action. Washington, DC: The National Academies Press, 2015.*

6. Miller GA. "The magical number seven plus or minus two: some limits on our capacity for processing information." *Psychol Rev.* Mar 1956; 63(2):81-97.

7. Mandell AM, Green RC. "Alzheimer's disease." In: Budson AE, Kowall NW, eds. *The handbook of Alzheimer's disease and other dementias.* Wiley-Blackwell; 2011:1-91:chap 1.

8. Boller F, Forbes MM. "History of dementia and dementia in history: an overview." *J Neurol Sci.* Jun 30

1998;158(2):125-33. doi:10.1016/s0022-510x (98)00128-2.

9. Mehta S. "Mild Cognitive Impairment." Medscape. 2019. https://emedicine.medscape.com/article/1136393 -overview. Accessed May 26, 2020.

10. Luo L, Craik FI. "Aging and memory: a cognitive approach." *Can J Psychiatry*. Jun 2008;53(6):346-53. doi:10.1177/070674370805300603.

11. Wellman M. "The concept of normal in medicine." *Can Med Assoc J*. Jul 1 1958;79(1):43-4.

12. Ge S, McConnell ES, Wu B, Pan W, Dong X, Plassman BL. "Longitudinal Association Between Hearing Loss, Vision Loss, Dual Sensory Loss, and Cognitive Decline." *J Am Geriatr Soc*. Mar 2021;69(3):644-650. doi:10.1111 /jgs.16933.

13. Kuo P-L, Huang AR, Ehrlich JR, et al. "Prevalence of Concurrent Functional Vision and Hearing Impairment and Association With Dementia in Community-Dwelling Medicare Beneficiaries." *JAMA Network Open*. 2021;4(3):e211558-e211558. doi:10.1001 /jamanetworkopen.2021.1558.

14. Wolski L, Leroi I, Regan J, et al. "The need for improved cognitive, hearing and vision assessments for older people with cognitive impairment: a qualitative study." *BMC Geriatr*. Dec 3 2019;19(1):328. doi:10.1186 /s12877-019-1336-3.

15. Mahmoudi E. "Hearing, Vision, or Dual Sensory Impairment and Dementia Risk." *JAMA Netw Open*. Mar 1 2021;4(3):e211846. doi:10.1001/jamanetworkopen .2021.1846.

16. Michalowsky B, Hoffmann W, Kostev K. "Association Between Hearing and Vision Impairment and Risk of Dementia: Results of a Case-Control Study Based

on Secondary Data." *Front Aging Neurosci.* 2019;11:363. doi:10.3389/fnagi.2019.00363.

17. Budson AE, Solomon PR. "Approach to the Patient with Memory Loss, Mild Cognitive Impairment, or Dementia." *Memory Loss, Alzheimer's Disease, and Dementia.* 2nd Edition ed. Elsevier; 2016:39-45:chap 3.

18. Critchley M. "The Neurology of Old Age." *Lancet.* 1931;217(5623):1221-1230.

19. Arnold SE. "'Senior Moments' or More? Diagnostic Evaluation of Cognitive Complaints in Older Adults and the Role of Cerebrospinal Fluid Biomarkers." *J Appl Lab Med.* Jan 1 2020;5(1):219-224. doi:10.1373/jalm.2019.029546.

20. Small GW. "What we need to know about age related memory loss." *BMJ.* Jun 22 2002;324(7352):1502-5. doi:10.1136/bmj.324.7352.1502.

21. Stanton BR. "The neurology of old age." *Clin Med (Lond).* Feb 2011;11(1):54-6. doi:10.7861/clinmedicine.11-1-54.

22. Buckley RF, Saling MM, Frommann I, Wolfsgruber S, Wagner M. "Subjective Cognitive Decline from a Phenomenological Perspective: A Review of the Qualitative Literature." *J Alzheimers Dis.* Sep 24 2015;48 Suppl 1:S125-40. doi:10.3233/JAD-150095.

23. Marais A. *Alzheimer's—or just senior moments?* Plus 502015. p. 16-17.

24. Smith M, Robinson L, Segal R. "Age-Related Memory Loss," 2019. *https://wwwhelpguideorg/articles/alzheimers-dementia-aging/age-related-memory-losshtm?pdf=12424. Accessed May 24, 2020.

25. Schott JM. "The neurology of ageing: what is normal?" *Pract Neurol.* Jun 2017;17(3):172-182. doi:10.1136/practneurol-2016-001566.

26. Naveh-Benjamin M, Mayr U. "Age-related differences in associative memory: Empirical evidence and theoretical

perspectives." *Psychol Aging*. Feb 2018;33(1):1-6. doi:10.1037/pag0000235.

27. Petersen R, Graff-Radford J. "Alzheimer's Disease and Other Dementias." *Bradley and Daroff's Neurology in Clinical Practice,*. Eighth ed. Elsevier; 2022:1452-1497:chap 95.

28. Murman DL. "The Impact of Age on Cognition." *Semin Hear*. Aug 2015;36(3):111-21. doi:10.1055/s-0035 -1555115.

29. Centers for Disease Control and Prevention (2019): "Subjective Cognitive Decline — A Public Health Issue" *Available from* https://wwwcdcgov/aging/data /subjective-cognitive-decline-briefhtml Accessed March 10, 2020.

30. Harrington KD, Schembri A, Lim YY, et al. "Estimates of age-related memory decline are inflated by unrecognized Alzheimer's disease." *Neurobiol Aging*. Oct 2018;70:170-179. doi:10.1016/j. neurobiolaging.2018.06.005.

31. Jessen F, Amariglio RE, van Boxtel M, et al. "A conceptual framework for research on subjective cognitive decline in preclinical Alzheimer's disease." *Alzheimers Dement*. Nov 2014;10(6):844-52. doi:10.1016/j .jalz.2014.01.001.

32. Jessen F, Amariglio RE, Buckley RF, et al. "The characterisation of subjective cognitive decline." *Lancet Neurol*. Mar 2020;19(3):271-278. doi:10.1016 /S1474-4422(19)30368-0.

33. Taylor CA, Bouldin ED, McGuire LC. "Subjective Cognitive Decline Among Adults Aged ≥45 Years - United States, 2015-2016." *MMWR Morb Mortal Wkly Rep*. Jul 13 2018;67(27):753-757. doi:10.15585/mmwr. mm6727a1.

34. Schneck MK, Reisberg B, Ferris SH. "An overview of current concepts of Alzheimer's disease." *Am J Psychiatry.* Feb 1982;139(2):165-73. doi:10.1176/ajp.139.2.165.

35. Reisberg B, Shao Y, Moosavi M, et al. "Psychometric Cognitive Decline Precedes the Advent of Subjective Cognitive Decline in the Evolution of Alzheimer's Disease." *Dement Geriatr Cogn Disord.* 2020;49(1):16-21. doi:10.1159/000507286.

36. Reisberg B, Ferris SH, de Leon MJ, et al. "Stage-specific behavioral, cognitive, and in vivo changes in community residing subjects with age-associated memory impairment and primary degenerative dementia of the Alzheimer type." *Drug Development Research.* 1988;15(2-3):101–114.

37. Reisberg B, Prichep L, Mosconi L, et al. "The pre-mild cognitive impairment, subjective cognitive impairment stage of Alzheimer's disease." *Alzheimers Dement.* Jan 2008;4(1 Suppl 1):S98-S108. doi:10.1016/j.jalz.2007.11.017.

38. Lenehan ME, Klekociuk SZ, Summers MJ. "Absence of a relationship between subjective memory complaint and objective memory impairment in mild cognitive impairment (MCI): is it time to abandon subjective memory complaint as an MCI diagnostic criterion?" *Int Psychogeriatr.* Sep 2012;24(9):1505-14. doi:10.1017/S1041610212000695.

39. Edmonds EC, Delano-Wood L, Galasko DR, Salmon DP, Bondi MW, "Alzheimer's Disease Neuroimaging I. Subjective cognitive complaints contribute to misdiagnosis of mild cognitive impairment." *Journal of the International Neuropsychological Society : JINS.* Sep 2014;20(8):836-47. doi:10.1017/S135561771400068X.

40. Jessen F, Wolfsgruber S, Kleineindam L, et al. "Subjective cognitive decline and stage 2 of Alzheimer disease in patients from memory centers." *Alzheimers Dement.* Apr 22 2022; doi:10.1002/alz.12674.

41. Miebach L, Wolfsgruber S, Polcher A, et al. "Which features of subjective cognitive decline are related to amyloid pathology? Findings from the DELCODE study." *Alzheimers Res Ther.* Jul 31 2019;11(1):66. doi:10.1186/s13195-019-0515-y.

42. Schütz H, Caspers S, Moebus S, Lux S. "Prevalence and psychosocial correlates of subjectively perceived decline in five cognitive domains: Results from a population-based cohort study in Germany." *Int J Geriatr Psychiatry.* Oct 2020;35(10):1219-1227. doi:10.1002/gps.5359

43. Budson A, Solomon P. *Memory loss, alzheimer's disease and dementia.* 3. ed. Elsevier, Inc; 2022:pages cm.

44. *ICD-10 : International statistical classification of diseases and related health problems: tenth revision. https://apps.who.int /iris/handle/10665/42980* . World Health Organization; 2004. https://apps.who.int/iris/handle/10665/42980.

45. Reisberg B, Shao Y, Moosavi M, et al. "Psychometric Cognitive Decline Precedes the Advent of Subjective Cognitive Decline in the Evolution of Alzheimer's Disease." *Dement Geriatr Cogn Disord.* 2020;49(1):16-21. doi:10.1159/000507286.

46. World Health Organization. (2004). ICD-10 : "International statistical classification of diseases and related health problems: tenth revision, 2nd ed." World Health Organization: Geneva. https://apps.who.int /iris/handle/10665/42980.

47. Sewell M, Li C, Sano M. "Neuropsychology in the Diagnosis and Treatment of Dementia." In: Fillit H, Rockwood K, Young J, eds. *Brocklehurst's textbook*

of geriatric medicine and gerontology. Eighth edition. ed. Elsevier, Inc.; 2017:389-397:chap 51.

48. Budson A, Solomon P. *Memory loss, alzheimer's disease and dementia*. 2 ed. Elsevier, Inc; 2016.

49. Jack CR, Jr., Bennett DA, Blennow K, et al. NIA-AA "Research Framework: Toward a biological definition of Alzheimer's disease." *Alzheimers Dement*. Apr 2018;14(4):535-562. doi:10.1016/j.jalz.2018.02.018.

50. Yu H, Wang K, Zhong P, Cheng HD, Lv XY, Yuan LL. "Investigations of Memory Monitoring in Individuals With Subjective Cognitive Decline and Amnestic Mild Cognitive Impairment." *Cogn Behav Neurol*. Sep 2020;33(3):201-207. doi:10.1097/wnn.00000000 00000242.

51. Gray DP, Dineen M, Sidaway-Lee K. "The worried well." *Br J Gen Pract*. Feb 2020;70(691):84-85. doi:10.3399/bjgp20X708017.

52. Jongsiriyanyong S, Limpawattana P. "Mild Cognitive Impairment in Clinical Practice: A Review Article." *Am J Alzheimers Dis Other Demen*. Dec 2018;33(8):500-507. doi:10.1177/1533317518791401.

53. Slot RER, Verfaillie SCJ, Overbeek JM, et al. "Subjective Cognitive Impairment Cohort (SCIENCe): study design and first results." *Alzheimers Res Ther*. Aug 7 2018;10(1):76. doi:10.1186/s13195-018-0390-y.

54. Studart AN, Nitrini R. "Subjective cognitive decline: The first clinical manifestation of Alzheimer's disease?" *Dement Neuropsychol*. Jul-Sep 2016;10(3):170-177. doi:10.1590/S1980-5764-2016DN1003002.

55. Scheltens P, Blennow K, Breteler MM, et al. "Alzheimer's disease." *Lancet*. Jul 30 2016;388(10043):505-17. doi:10.1016/s0140-6736(15)01124-1.

56. Miebach L, Wolfsgruber S, Polcher A, et al. "Which features of subjective cognitive decline are related to

amyloid pathology? Findings from the DELCODE study." *Alzheimers Res Ther.* Jul 31 2019;11(1):66. doi:10.1186/s13195-019-0515-y.

57. Molinuevo JL, Rabin LA, Amariglio R, et al. "Implementation of subjective cognitive decline criteria in research studies." *Alzheimers Dement.* Mar 2017;13(3):296-311. doi:10.1016/j.jalz.2016.09.012.

58. Dubois B, Hampel H, Feldman HH, et al. "Preclinical Alzheimer's disease: Definition, natural history, and diagnostic criteria." *Alzheimers Dement.* Mar 2016;12(3):292-323. doi:10.1016/j.jalz.2016.02.002.

59. Yeh TS, Yuan C, Ascherio A, Rosner B, Willett W, Blacker D. "Long-term Dietary Flavonoid Intake and Subjective Cognitive Decline in US Men and Women." *Neurology.* Jul 28 2021. doi:10.1212/WNL.000000000 0012454.

60. Yuan C, Fondell E, Bhushan A, et al. "Long-term intake of vegetables and fruits and subjective cognitive function in US men." *Neurology.* Jan 1 2019;92(1):e63-e75. doi:10.1212/WNL.0000000000006684.

61. Rabin LA, Smart CM, Amariglio RE. "Subjective Cognitive Decline in Preclinical Alzheimer's Disease." *Annu Rev Clin Psychol.* May 8 2017;13:369-396. doi:10.1146/annurev-clinpsy-032816-045136.

62. Rami L, Mollica MA, Garcia-Sanchez C, et al. "The Subjective Cognitive Decline Questionnaire (SCD-Q): a validation study." *J Alzheimers Dis.* 2014;41(2):453-66. doi:10.3233/JAD-132027.

63. Valech N, Mollica MA, Olives J, et al. "Informants' Perception of Subjective Cognitive Decline Helps to Discriminate Preclinical Alzheimer's Disease from Normal Aging." *J Alzheimers Dis.* Sep 24 2015;48 Suppl 1:S87-98. doi:10.3233/jad-150117.

64. Taler V, Morrison C, Sheppard C. "Cognitive Performance in Older Adults With Subjective Cognitive Decline." *Innovation in Aging*. 2020;4(1):291.

65. Gatchel JR, Wright CI, Falk WE, Trinh N. "Dementia." In: Stern TA, ed. *Massachusetts General Hospital comprehensive clinical psychiatry*. 2nd ed. Mosby/Elsevier; 2016:184-197:chap 19.

66. Janssen O, Jansen WJ, Vos SJB, et al. "Characteristics of subjective cognitive decline associated with amyloid positivity." *Alzheimers Dement*. Dec 8 2021. doi:10.1002/alz.12512.

67. Valech N, Sánchez-Benavides G, Tort-Merino A, et al. "Associations Between the Subjective Cognitive Decline-Questionnaire's Scores, Gray Matter Volume, and Amyloid-β Levels." *J Alzheimers Dis*. 2019;72(4):1287-1302. doi:10.3233/jad-190624.

68. Peter J, Scheef L, Abdulkadir A, et al. "Gray matter atrophy pattern in elderly with subjective memory impairment." *Alzheimers Dement*. Jan 2014;10(1):99-108. doi:10.1016/j.jalz.2013.05.1764.

69. Eliassen CF, Reinvang I, Selnes P, Grambaite R, Fladby T, Hessen E. "Biomarkers in subtypes of mild cognitive impairment and subjective cognitive decline." *Brain Behav*. Sep 2017;7(9):e00776. doi:10.1002/brb3.776.

70. Dubois B, Feldman HH, Jacova C, et al. Advancing research diagnostic criteria for Alzheimer's disease: the IWG-2 criteria. *Lancet Neurol*. Jun 2014;13(6):614-29. doi:10.1016/S1474-4422(14)70090-0.

71. Lista S, Molinuevo JL, Cavedo E, et al. "Evolving Evidence for the Value of Neuroimaging Methods and Biological Markers in Subjects Categorized with Subjective Cognitive Decline." *J Alzheimers Dis*. Sep 24 2015;48 Suppl 1:S171-91. doi:10.3233/jad-150202.

72. Slot RER, Sikkes SAM, Berkhof J, et al. "Subjective cognitive decline and rates of incident Alzheimer's disease and non-Alzheimer's disease dementia." *Alzheimers Dement.* Mar 2019;15(3):465-476. doi:10.1016/j .jalz.2018.10.003.

73. Desai AK, Schwarz L. "Subjective cognitive impairment: When to be concerned about 'senior moments.'" *Current Psychiatry.* 2011;10(4):21-35.

74. Lee YM, Ha JK, Park JM, et al. "Impact of Apolipoprotein E4 Polymorphism on the Gray Matter Volume and the White Matter Integrity in Subjective Memory Impairment without White Matter Hyperintensities: Voxel-Based Morphometry and Tract-Based Spatial Statistics Study under 3-Tesla MRI." *J Neuroimaging.* Jan-Feb 2016;26(1):144-9. doi:10.1111 /jon.12207.

75. Dik MG, Jonker C, Comijs HC, et al. "Memory complaints and APOE-epsilon4 accelerate cognitive decline in cognitively normal elderly." *Neurology.* Dec 26 2001;57(12):2217-22. doi:10.1212/wnl.57.12.2217.

76. Samieri C, Proust-Lima C, M MG, et al. "Subjective cognitive concerns, episodic memory, and the APOE epsilon4 allele." *Alzheimers Dement.* Nov 2014;10(6):752-759 e1. doi:10.1016/j.jalz.2014.06.012.

77. Krell-Roesch J, Woodruff BK, Acosta JI, et al. "APOE ε4 Genotype and the Risk for Subjective Cognitive Impairment in Elderly Persons." *J Neuropsychiatry Clin Neurosci.* Fall 2015;27(4):322-5. doi:10.1176/appi. neuropsych.14100268.

78. Mosconi L, De Santi S, Brys M, et al. "Hypometabolism and altered cerebrospinal fluid markers in normal apolipoprotein E E4 carriers with subjective memory complaints." *Biol Psychiatry.* Mar 15 2008;63(6):609-18. doi:10.1016/j.biopsych.2007.05.030.

79. Rowe CC, Ellis KA, Rimajova M, et al. "Amyloid imaging results from the Australian Imaging, Biomarkers and Lifestyle (AIBL) study of aging." *Neurobiol Aging*. Aug 2010;31(8):1275-83. doi:10.1016/j.neurobiolaging.2010.04.007.

80. Zwan MD, Villemagne VL, Doré V, et al. "Subjective Memory Complaints in APOEε4 Carriers are Associated with High Amyloid-β Burden." *J Alzheimers Dis*. 2016;49(4):1115-22. doi:10.3233/jad-150446.

81. Stewart R, Godin O, Crivello F, et al. "Longitudinal neuroimaging correlates of subjective memory impairment: 4-year prospective community study." *Br J Psychiatry*. Mar 2011;198(3):199-205. doi:10.1192/bjp.bp.110.078683.

82. Striepens N, Scheef L, Wind A, et al. "Interaction effects of subjective memory impairment and ApoE4 genotype on episodic memory and hippocampal volume." *Psychol Med*. Sep 2011;41(9):1997-2006. doi:10.1017/s0033291711000067.

83. Mendonca MD, Alves L, Bugalho P. "From Subjective Cognitive Complaints to Dementia: Who is at Risk?: A Systematic Review." *Am J Alzheimers Dis Other Demen*. Mar 2016;31(2):105-14. doi:10.1177/1533317515592331.

84. Westoby CJ, Mallen CD, Thomas E. "Cognitive complaints in a general population of older adults: prevalence, association with pain and the influence of concurrent affective disorders." *Eur J Pain*. Oct 2009;13(9):970-6. doi:10.1016/j.ejpain.2008.11.011.

85. Luck T, Roehr S, Rodriguez FS, et al. "Memory-related subjective cognitive symptoms in the adult population: prevalence and associated factors - results of the LIFE-Adult-Study." *BMC Psychol*. May 21 2018;6(1):23. doi:10.1186/s40359-018-0236-1.

86. Zullo L, Clark C, Gholam M, et al. "Factors associated with subjective cognitive decline in dementia-free older adults-A population-based study." *Int J Geriatr Psychiatry*. Aug 2021;36(8):1188-1196. doi:10.1002/gps.5509

87. Alzheimer's Association National Plan C, Support Milestone; Borson S, et al. "Report on milestones for care and support under the U.S. National Plan to Address Alzheimer's Disease." *Alzheimers Dement*. Mar 2016;12(3):334-69. doi:10.1016/j.jalz.2016.01.005.

88. Jonker C, Geerlings MI, Schmand B. "Are memory complaints predictive for dementia? A review of clinical and population-based studies." *Int J Geriatr Psychiatry*. Nov 2000;15(11):983-91. doi:10.1002/1099-1166(200011)15:11<983::aid-gps238>3.0.co;2-5.

89. Si T, Xing G, Han Y. "Subjective Cognitive Decline and Related Cognitive Deficits." *Front Neurol*. 2020;11:247. doi:10.3389/fneur.2020.00247.

90. Jeffers EM, Bouldin ED, McGuire LC, et al. "Prevalence and Characteristics of Subjective Cognitive Decline Among Unpaid Caregivers Aged >/=45 Years - 22 States, 2015-2019." *MMWR Morb Mortal Wkly Rep*. Nov 19 2021;70(46):1591-1596. doi:10.15585/mmwr.mm7046a1.

91. Wen C, Hu H, Ou YN, et al. "Risk factors for subjective cognitive decline: the CABLE study." *Transl Psychiatry*. Nov 9 2021;11(1):576. doi:10.1038/s41398-021-01711-1.

92. Jessen F, Amariglio RE, van Boxtel M, et al. "A conceptual framework for research on subjective cognitive decline in preclinical Alzheimer's disease." *Alzheimers Dement*. Nov 2014;10(6):844-52. doi:10.1016/j.jalz.2014.01.001.

93. Jessen F, Amariglio RE, van Boxtel M, et al. "A conceptual framework for research on subjective cognitive decline in preclinical Alzheimer's disease." *Alzheimers Dement.* Nov 2014;10(6):844-52. doi:10.1016/j.jalz.2014.01.001.

94. Pavisic IM, Lu K, Keuss SE, et al. "Subjective cognitive complaints at age 70: associations with amyloid and mental health." *J Neurol Neurosurg Psychiatry.* Nov 2021;92(11):1215-1221. doi:10.1136/jnnp-2020-325620.

95. Sutherland M, Kirk A, Karunanayake CP, O'Connell ME, Morgan DG. "What Happens to the Worried Well? Follow-Up of Subjective Cognitive Impairment." *Can J Neurol Sci.* Jan 2022;49(1):84-92. doi:10.1017/cjn.2021.39.

96. Rodriguez-Gomez O, Abdelnour C, Jessen F, Valero S, Boada M. "Influence of Sampling and Recruitment Methods in Studies of Subjective Cognitive Decline." *J Alzheimers Dis.* Sep 24 2015;48 Suppl 1:S99-S107. doi:10.3233/JAD-150189.

97. Curhan SG, Willett WC, Grodstein F, Curhan GC. "Longitudinal study of hearing loss and subjective cognitive function decline in men." *Alzheimers Dement.* Apr 2019;15(4):525-533. doi:10.1016/j.jalz.2018.11.004.

98. Mallo SC, Ismail Z, Pereiro AX, et al. "Assessing Mild Behavioral Impairment with the Mild Behavioral Impairment-Checklist in People with Mild Cognitive Impairment." *J Alzheimers Dis.* 2018;66(1):83-95. doi:10.3233/JAD-180131.

99. van Oijen M, de Jong FJ, Hofman A, Koudstaal PJ, Breteler MM. "Subjective memory complaints, education, and risk of Alzheimer's disease."

Alzheimers Dement. Apr 2007;3(2):92-7. doi:10.1016/j. jalz.2007.01.011.

100. Mitchell AJ, Beaumont H, Ferguson D, Yadegarfar M, Stubbs B. "Risk of dementia and mild cognitive impairment in older people with subjective memory complaints: meta-analysis." *Acta Psychiatr Scand.* Dec 2014;130(6):439-51. doi:10.1111/acps.12336.

101. Reisberg B, Shulman MB, Torossian C, Leng L, Zhu W. "Outcome over seven years of healthy adults with and without subjective cognitive impairment." *Alzheimers Dement.* Jan 2010;6(1):11-24. doi:10.1016/j .jalz.2009.10.002.

102. Schwilk N, Kloppel S, Schmidtke K, Metternich B. "Functional cognitive disorder in subjective cognitive decline—A 10-year follow-up." *Int J Geriatr Psychiatry.* May 2021;36(5):677-683. doi:10.1002/gps.5466.

103. Kaup AR, Nettiksimmons J, LeBlanc ES, Yaffe K. "Memory complaints and risk of cognitive impairment after nearly 2 decades among older women." *Neurology.* Nov 24 2015;85(21):1852-8. doi:10.1212 /wnl.0000000000002153.

104. Pike KE, Ellis KA, Villemagne VL, et al. "Cognition and beta-amyloid in preclinical Alzheimer's disease: data from the AIBL study." *Neuropsychologia.* Jul 2011;49(9):2384-90. doi:10.1016/j. neuropsychologia.2011.04.012.

105. Rabin LA, Wang C, Mogle JA, Lipton RB, Derby CA, Katz MJ. "An approach to classifying subjective cognitive decline in community-dwelling elders." *Alzheimers Dement (Amst).* 2020;12(1):e12103. doi:10.1002/dad2.12103.

106. Lyketsos CG, Carrillo MC, Ryan JM, et al. "Neuropsychiatric symptoms in Alzheimer's disease."

Alzheimers Dement. Sep 2011;7(5):532-9. doi:10.1016/j .jalz.2011.05.2410.

107. Masters MC, Morris JC, Roe CM. "'Noncognitive' symptoms of early Alzheimer disease: a longitudinal analysis." *Neurology.* Feb 10 2015;84(6):617-22. doi:10.1212/wnl.0000000000001238.

108. Jessen F, Wiese B, Bachmann C, et al. "Prediction of dementia by subjective memory impairment: effects of severity and temporal association with cognitive impairment." *Arch Gen Psychiatry.* Apr 2010;67(4):414-22. doi:10.1001/archgenpsychiatry.2010.30.

109. Hessen E, Eckerström M, Nordlund A, et al. "Subjective Cognitive Impairment Is a Predominantly Benign Condition in Memory Clinic Patients Followed for 6 Years: The Gothenburg-Oslo MCI Study." *Dement Geriatr Cogn Dis Extra.* Jan-Apr 2017;7(1):1-14. doi:10.1159/000454676.

110. van Harten AC, Visser PJ, Pijnenburg YA, et al. "Cerebrospinal fluid Aβ42 is the best predictor of clinical progression in patients with subjective complaints." *Alzheimers Dement.* Sep 2013;9(5):481-7. doi:10.1016/j .jalz.2012.08.004.

111. Rubin R. "Neurologist Faces His Alzheimer Diagnosis Determined to Lessen Stigma Surrounding the Disease." *JAMA.* Apr 28 2021. doi:10.1001/jama.2021.5333.

112. Reisberg B, Gauthier S. "Current evidence for subjective cognitive impairment (SCI) as the pre-mild cognitive impairment (MCI) stage of subsequently manifest Alzheimer's disease." *Int Psychogeriatr.* Feb 2008;20(1): 1-16. doi:10.1017/S1041610207006412.

113. Bhome R, Berry AJ, Huntley JD, Howard RJ. "Interventions for subjective cognitive decline:

systematic review and meta-analysis." *BMJ Open*. Jul 19 2018;8(7):e021610. doi:10.1136/bmjopen-2018-021610.

114. Roheger M, Hennersdorf XS, Riemann S, Floel A, Meinzer M. "A systematic review and network meta-analysis of interventions for subjective cognitive decline." *Alzheimers Dement (N Y)*. 2021;7(1):e12180. doi:10.1002 /trc2.12180.

115. Livingston G, Huntley J, Sommerlad A, et al. "Dementia prevention, intervention, and care: 2020 report of the Lancet Commission." *Lancet*. Aug 8 2020;396(10248):413-446. doi:10.1016 /S0140-6736(20)30367-6.

116. Chun CT, Seward K, Patterson A, Melton A, MacDonald-Wicks L. "Evaluation of Available Cognitive Tools Used to Measure Mild Cognitive Decline: A Scoping Review." *Nutrients*. Nov 8 2021;13(11). doi:10.3390/nu13113974.

117. "2021 Alzheimer's disease facts and figures." *Alzheimers Dement*. Mar 2021;17(3):327-406. doi:10.1002 /alz.12328.

118. Reisberg B, Ferris SH, de Leon MJ, Crook T. "The Global Deterioration Scale for assessment of primary degenerative dementia." *Am J Psychiatry*. Sep 1982;139(9):1136-9. doi:10.1176/ajp.139.9.1136.

119. Allen M, Zou F, Chai HS, et al. "Novel late-onset Alzheimer disease loci variants associate with brain gene expression." *Neurology*. Jul 17 2012;79(3):221-8. doi:10.1212/WNL.0b013e3182605801.

120. Reisberg B, Torossian C, Shulman MB, et al. "Two-Year Outcomes, Cognitive and Behavioral Markers of Decline in Healthy, Cognitively Normal Older Persons with Global Deterioration Scale Stage 2 (Subjective

Cognitive Decline with Impairment)." *J Alzheimers Dis.* 2019;67(2):685-705. doi:10.3233/JAD-180341.

121. Reisberg B. "Functional assessment staging (FAST)." *Psychopharmacol Bull.* 1988;24(4):653-9.

122. Buckley RF, Saling MM, Frommann I, Wolfsgruber S, Wagner M. "Subjective Cognitive Decline from a Phenomenological Perspective: A Review of the Qualitative Literature." *J Alzheimers Dis.* Sep 24 2015;48 Suppl 1:S125-40. doi:10.3233/JAD-150095.

123. Petersen RC. "Clinical practice. Mild cognitive impairment." *N Engl J Med.* Jun 09 2011;364(23):2227-34. doi:10.1056/NEJMcp0910237.

124. Budson AE, Solomon PR. "Subjective Cognitive Decline, Mild Cognitive Impairment, and Dementia." *Memory Loss, Alzheimer's Disease and Dementia.* 3 ed. Elsevier; 2022:28-47:chap 3.

125. Alzheimer disease. *Clinical Overview Clinical Key.* Updated June 14, 2018. Accessed May 10, 2019.

126. Brown AS. "A review of the tip-of-the-tongue experience." *Psychol Bull.* Mar 1991;109(2):204-23. doi:10.1037/0033-2909.109.2.204.

127. Brown AS. *The Tip of the Tongue State.* Psychology Press; 2012.

128. Brown R, McNeill D. "The "tip of the tongue" phenomenon." *Journal of Verbal Learning & Verbal Behavior.* 1966;5(4):325-337. doi:https://psycnet.apa.org/doi/10.1016/S0022-5371(66)80040-3.

129. Juncos-Rabadan O, Facal D, Pereiro AX. "Tip-of-the-tongue in Mild cognitive impairment (MCI)." In: Schwartz BL, Brown AS, eds. *Tip-of-the-Tongue States and Related Phenomena.* Cambridge University Press; 2014:116-143:chap 7.

130. Campos-Magdaleno M, Leiva D, Pereiro AX, et al. "Longitudinal Patterns of the Tip-of-the-Tongue Phenomenon in People With Subjective Cognitive Complaints and Mild Cognitive Impairment." *Front Psychol.* 2020;11:425. doi:10.3389/fpsyg.2020.00425.

131. Juncos-Rabadan O, Facal D, Lojo-Seoane C, Pereiro AX. "Does tip-of-the-tongue for proper names discriminate amnestic mild cognitive impairment?" *Int Psychogeriatr.* Apr 2013;25(4):627-34. doi:10.1017/S1041610212002207.

132. Abrams L, Davis D. "The tip-of-the-tongue phenomenon: Who, what, and why." In: Wright HH, ed. *Cognition, language and aging.* John Benjamins Publishing Company; 2016:13-53:chap 2.

133. Jack CR, Jr., Bennett DA, Blennow K, et al. "NIA-AA Research Framework: Toward a biological definition of Alzheimer's disease." *Alzheimers Dement.* Apr 2018;14(4):535-562. doi:10.1016/j.jalz.2018.02.018.

134. American Psychiatric Association. *Diagnostic and statistical manual of mental disorders : DSM-5-TR.* Fifth edition, text revision. ed. American Psychiatric Association Publishing; 2022:lxix, 1050 pages.

135. Chun CT, Seward K, Patterson A, Melton A, MacDonald-Wicks L. "Evaluation of Available Cognitive Tools Used to Measure Mild Cognitive Decline: A Scoping Review." *Nutrients.* Nov 8 2021;13(11). doi:10.3390/nu13113974.

136. Molinuevo JL, Rabin LA, Amariglio R, et al. "Implementation of subjective cognitive decline criteria in research studies." *Alzheimers Dement.* Mar 2017;13(3):296-311. doi:10.1016/j.jalz.2016.09.012.

137. Maruff P, Lim YY, Darby D, et al. "Clinical utility of the cogstate brief battery in identifying cognitive

impairment in mild cognitive impairment and Alzheimer's disease." *BMC Psychol.* 2013;1(1):30. doi:10.1186/2050-7283-1-30.

138. Bruno D, Schurmann Vignaga S. "Addenbrooke's cognitive examination III in the diagnosis of dementia: a critical review." *Neuropsychiatr Dis Treat.* 2019;15:441-447. doi:10.2147/NDT.S151253.

139. Brown JM, Lansdall CJ, Wiggins J, et al. "The Test Your Memory for Mild Cognitive Impairment (TYM-MCI)." *J Neurol Neurosurg Psychiatry.* Dec 2017;88(12):1045-1051. doi:10.1136/jnnp-2016-315327.

140. Potts C, Richardson J, Bond RB, et al. "Reliability of Addenbrooke's Cognitive Examination III in differentiating between dementia, mild cognitive impairment and older adults who have not reported cognitive problems." *Eur J Ageing.* Sep 22 2021:1-13. doi:10.1007/s10433-021-00652-4.

141. Terpening Z, Cordato NJ, Hepner IJ, Lucas SK, Lindley RI. "Utility of the Addenbrooke's Cognitive Examination—Revised for the diagnosis of dementia syndromes." *Australas J Ageing.* Sep 2011;30(3):113-8. doi:10.1111/j.1741-6612.2010.00446.x

142. Abner EL, Kryscio RJ, Caban-Holt AM, Schmitt FA. "Baseline subjective memory complaints associate with increased risk of incident dementia: the PREADVISE trial." *J Prev Alzheimers Dis.* Mar 2015;2(1):11-16. doi:10.14283/jpad.2015.37.

143. Brown JM, Wiggins J, Dong H, et al. "The hard Test Your Memory. Evaluation of a short cognitive test to detect mild Alzheimer's disease and amnestic mild cognitive impairment." *Int J Geriatr Psychiatry.* Mar 2014;29(3):272-80. doi:10.1002/gps.4005.

144. Brown JM, Wiggins J, Dawson K, Rittman T, Rowe JB. "Test Your Memory (TYM) and Test Your Memory for

Mild Cognitive Impairment (TYM-MCI): A Review and Update Including Results of Using the TYM Test in a General Neurology Clinic and Using a Telephone Version of the TYM Test." *Diagnostics (Basel)*. Sep 8 2019;9(3). doi:10.3390/diagnostics9030116.

145. Scharre DW, Chang SI, Murden RA, et al. "Self-administered Gerocognitive Examination (SAGE): a brief cognitive assessment Instrument for mild cognitive impairment (MCI) and early dementia." *Alzheimer Dis Assoc Disord*. Jan-Mar 2010;24(1):64-71. doi:10.1097/WAD.0b013e3181b03277.

146. Scharre DW, Chang SI, Nagaraja HN, Wheeler NC, Kataki M. "Self-Administered Gerocognitive Examination: longitudinal cohort testing for the early detection of dementia conversion." *Alzheimers Res Ther*. Dec 6 2021;13(1):192. doi:10.1186/s13195-021-00930-4.

147. Goodman DM. "I Forget Names All the Time: Could This Be Alzheimer's Disease?" *Medscape*. Nov 24 2021. https://www.medscape.com/viewarticle/963519. Accessed February 14, 2022. 2021;

148. Niedźwieńska A, Kvavilashvili L. "Everyday Memory Failures in Older Adults with Amnestic Mild Cognitive Impairment." *J Alzheimers Dis*. 2019;70(1):257-275. doi:10.3233/jad-190219.

149. Petersen RC, Lopez O, Armstrong MJ, et al. "Practice guideline update summary: Mild cognitive impairment: Report of the Guideline Development, Dissemination, and Implementation Subcommittee of the American Academy of Neurology." *Neurology*. Jan 16 2018;90(3):126-135. doi:10.1212/WNL.0000000000004826.

150. Hale JM, Schneider DC, Mehta NK, Myrskyla M. "Cognitive impairment in the U.S.: Lifetime risk, age

at onset, and years impaired." *SSM Popul Health*. Aug 2020;11:100577. doi:10.1016/j.ssmph.2020.100577.

151. Petersen RC. "Mild Cognitive Impairment." *Continuum (Minneap Minn)*. Apr 2016;22(2 Dementia):404-18. doi:10.1212/CON.0000000000000313.

152. Yoneda T, Graham E, Lozinski T, et al. "Personality traits, cognitive states, and mortality in older adulthood." *J Pers Soc Psychol*. Apr 11 2022. doi:10.1037/pspp0000418.

153. Wang J, Wang L, Zhou X, Wen X, Zhen X. "Risk factors for predicting progression from normal cognition to mild cognitive impairment: protocol for a systematic review and meta-analysis of cohort studies." *BMJ Open*. Jun 11 2019;9(6):e027313. doi:10.1136/bmjopen-2018-027313.

154. Li JQ, Tan L, Wang HF, et al. "Risk factors for predicting progression from mild cognitive impairment to Alzheimer's disease: a systematic review and meta-analysis of cohort studies." *J Neurol Neurosurg Psychiatry*. May 2016;87(5):476-84. doi:10.1136/jnnp-2014-310095.

155. Visser PJ, Verhey F, Knol DL, et al. "Prevalence and prognostic value of CSF markers of Alzheimer's disease pathology in patients with subjective cognitive impairment or mild cognitive impairment in the DESCRIPA study: a prospective cohort study." *Lancet Neurol*. Jul 2009;8(7):619-27. doi:10.1016/S1474-4422(09)70139-5.

156. Sierra-Rio A, Balasa M, Olives J, et al. "Cerebrospinal Fluid Biomarkers Predict Clinical Evolution in Patients with Subjective Cognitive Decline and Mild Cognitive Impairment." *Neurodegener Dis*. 2016;16(1-2):69-76. doi:10.1159/000439258.

157. Holsinger T, Plassman BL, Stechuchak KM, Burke JR, Coffman CJ, Williams JW, Jr. "Stability of Diagnoses of Cognitive Impairment, Not Dementia in a Veterans Affairs Primary Care Population." *J Am Geriatr Soc.* Jun 2015;63(6):1105-11. doi:10.1111/jgs.13455.

158. Petersen RC. "Clinical practice. Mild cognitive impairment." *N Engl J Med.* Jun 9 2011;364(23):2227-34. doi:10.1056/NEJMcp0910237.

159. Hajjar I, Okafor M, McDaniel D, et al. "Effects of Candesartan vs Lisinopril on Neurocognitive Function in Older Adults With Executive Mild Cognitive Impairment: A Randomized Clinical Trial." *JAMA Netw Open.* Aug 3 2020;3(8):e2012252. doi:10.1001/jamanetworkopen.2020.12252.

160. National Academies of Sciences E, Medicine, Division of B, et al. "The National Academies Collection: Reports funded by National Institutes of Health." *Reducing the Impact of Dementia in America: A Decadal Survey of the Behavioral and Social Sciences.* National Academies Press (US), 2021.

161. National Academies of Sciences, Engineering, and Medicine. "Alzheimer's Disease and Related Dementias: Experience and Caregiving, Epidemiology, and Models of Care: Proceedings of a Workshop in Brief." Washington, DC: The National Academies Press, 2020. https://doi.org/10.17226/25694. https://www.nap.edu/catalog/25694/alzheimers-disease-and-related-dementias-experience-and-caregiving-epidemiology-and-models-of-care. Accessed August 2, 2020.

162. Murphy SL, Kochanek KD, Xu J, Arias E. "Mortality in the United States, 2020." *NCHS Data Brief.* Dec 2021;(427):1-8.

163. Global status report on the public health response to dementia. Geneva: World Health Organization, 2021.

164. Gatchel JR, Lopera F, Norton DJ, et al. "Association of subjective cognitive decline with markers of brain pathology in preclinical autosomal dominant Alzheimer's disease." *J Neurol Neurosurg Psychiatry*. Mar 2020;91(3):330-332. doi:10.1136/jnnp-2019-321205,

165. National Academies of Sciences, Engineering, and Medicine. "Challenging Questions about Epidemiology, Care, and Caregiving for People with Alzheimer's Disease and Related Dementias and Their Families: Proceedings of a Workshop in Brief." Washington, DC: The National Academies Press, 2020. https ://doi.org/10.17226/25706. https://www.nap.edu /catalog/25706/challenging-questions-about -epidemiology-care-and-caregiving-for-people-with -alzheimers-disease-and-related-dementias-and-their -families. Accessed August 2, 2020. 2020;

166. Hippius H, Neundorfer G. "The discovery of Alzheimer's disease." *Dialogues Clin Neurosci*. Mar 2003;5(1):101-8.

167. Silva MVF, Loures CMG, Alves LCV, de Souza LC, Borges KBG, Carvalho MDG. "Alzheimer's disease: risk factors and potentially protective measures." *J Biomed Sci*. May 9 2019;26(1):33. doi:10.1186/ s12929-019-0524-y.

168. Dubois B, Hampel H, Feldman HH, et al. "Preclinical Alzheimer's disease: Definition, natural history, and diagnostic criteria." *Alzheimers Dement*. Mar 2016;12(3):292-323. doi:10.1016/j.jalz.2016.02.002.

169. Budson AE, Solomon PR. "Special Issues in Memory Loss, Alzheimer's Disease, and Dementia." *Memory Loss,*

Alzheimer's Disease and Dementia. 3 ed. Elsevier; 2022:297-300:chap 30.

170. Shaw G. "Genetic Testing May Influence Treatment of Neurologic Disorders." *Brain&Life*, February/March 2022 https://www.brainandlife.org/articles/genetic-testing-influence-treatment-neurologic-disorders. Accessed May 7, 2022.

171. Seto M, Weiner RL, Dumitrescu L, Hohman TJ. "Protective genes and pathways in Alzheimer's disease: moving towards precision interventions." *Mol Neurodegener.* Apr 29 2021;16(1):29. doi:10.1186/s13024-021-00452-5.

172. Park DC, Festini SB. "Theories of Memory and Aging: A Look at the Past and a Glimpse of the Future." *J Gerontol B Psychol Sci Soc Sci.* Jan 2017;72(1):82-90. doi:10.1093/geronb/gbw066.

173. Mander BA, Winer JR, Walker MP. "Sleep and Human Aging." *Neuron.* Apr 5 2017;94(1):19-36. doi:10.1016/j.neuron.2017.02.004.

174. Nicholas LH, Langa KM, Bynum JPW, Hsu JW. "Financial Presentation of Alzheimer Disease and Related Dementias." *JAMA internal medicine.* Feb 1 2021;181(2):220-227. doi:10.1001/jamainternmed.2020.6432.

175. Eikelboom WS, van den Berg E, Singleton EH, et al. "Neuropsychiatric and Cognitive Symptoms Across the Alzheimer Disease Clinical Spectrum: Cross-sectional and Longitudinal Associations." *Neurology.* Sep 28 2021;97(13):e1276-e1287. doi:10.1212/wnl.0000000000012598.

176. Reisberg B, Ferris SH, de Leon MJ, Crook T. "The Global Deterioration Scale for assessment of

primary degenerative dementia." *Am J Psychiatry*. Sep 1982;139(9):1136-9. doi:10.1176/ajp.139.9.1136.

177. Reisberg B, Ferris SH, de Leon MJ, et al. "The stage specific temporal course of Alzheimer's disease: functional and behavioral concomitants based upon cross-sectional and longitudinal observation." *Prog Clin Biol Res*. 1989;317:23-41.

178. Reisberg B. Alzheimer's disease. "Stages of cognitive decline." *Am J Nurs*. Feb 1984;84(2):225-8.

179. Sperling RA, Aisen PS, Beckett LA, et al. "Toward defining the preclinical stages of Alzheimer's disease: recommendations from the National Institute on Aging-Alzheimer's Association workgroups on diagnostic guidelines for Alzheimer's disease." *Alzheimers Dement*. May 2011;7(3):280-92. doi:10.1016/j.jalz.2011.03.003.

180. *Risk Reduction of Cognitive Decline and Dementia: WHO Guidelines*. WHO Guidelines Approved by the Guidelines Review Committee, 2019.

181. WHO, World Health Organization. *Global action plan on the public health response to dementia, 2017–2025*. Geneva: World Health Organization, 2017.

182. Kane RL, Butler M, Fink HA, et al. "Interventions to Prevent Age-Related Cognitive Decline, Mild Cognitive Impairment, and Clinical Alzheimer's-Type Dementia." AHRQ Comparative Effectiveness Reviews, 2017.

183. National Academies of Sciences, Engineering, and Medicine. *Preventing Cognitive Decline and Dementia: A Way Forward*. The National Academies Press, 2017.

184. Bennett DA, Wilson RS, Boyle PA, Buchman AS, Schneider JA. "Relation of neuropathology to cognition in persons without cognitive impairment." *Ann Neurol*. Oct 2012;72(4):599-609. doi:10.1002/ana.23654.

185. Monsell SE, Mock C, Hassenstab J, et al. "Neuropsychological changes in asymptomatic persons with Alzheimer disease neuropathology." *Neurology.* Jul 29 2014;83(5):434-40. doi:10.1212/wnl.00000000 00000650.

186. Hubbard BM, Fenton GW, Anderson JM. "A quantitative histological study of early clinical and preclinical Alzheimer's disease." *Neuropathol Appl Neurobiol.* Apr 1990;16(2):111-21. doi:10.1111/j.1365-2990.1990. tb00940.x.

187. Jansen WJ, Ossenkoppele R, Knol DL, et al. "Prevalence of cerebral amyloid pathology in persons without dementia: a meta-analysis." *JAMA.* May 19 2015;313(19):1924-38. doi:10.1001/jama.2015.4668.

188. Vos SJ, Xiong C, Visser PJ, et al. "Preclinical Alzheimer's disease and its outcome: a longitudinal cohort study." *Lancet Neurol.* Oct 2013;12(10):957-65. doi:10.1016 /s1474-4422(13)70194-7.

189. Hansson O, Blennow K, Zetterberg H, Dage J. "Blood biomarkers for Alzheimer's disease in clinical practice and trials." *Nat Aging.* May 2023;3(5):506-519. doi:10.1038/s43587-023-00403-3.

190. van der Flier WM, de Vugt ME, Smets EMA, Blom M, Teunissen CE. "Towards a future where Alzheimer's disease pathology is stopped before the onset of dementia." *Nat Aging.* May 2023;3(5):494-505. doi:10.1038/s43587-023-00404-2.

191. National Academies of Sciences E, Medicine, Division of B, et al. "The National Academies Collection: Reports funded by National Institutes of Health." In: Forstag EH, ed. *Implications for Behavioral and Social Research of Preclinical Markers of Alzheimer's Disease and*

Related Dementias: Proceedings of a Workshop—in Brief. National Academies Press (US), 2021.

192. Sperling RA, Karlawish J, Johnson KA. "Preclinical Alzheimer disease—the challenges ahead." *Nat Rev Neurol.* Jan 2013;9(1):54-8. doi:10.1038/nrneurol.2012.241.

193. Pettigrew C, Soldan A, Wang J, et al. "Longitudinal CSF Alzheimer's disease biomarker changes from middle age to late adulthood." *Alzheimer's & Dementia: Diagnosis, Assessment & Disease Monitoring.* 2022;14(1):e12374. doi:https://doi.org/10.1002/dad2.12374.

194. Hohman TJ, Dumitrescu L, Cox NJ, Jefferson AL, "Alzheimer's Neuroimaging I. Genetic resilience to amyloid related cognitive decline." *Brain Imaging Behav.* Apr 2017;11(2):401-409. doi:10.1007/s11682-016-9615-5.

195. Begley S. "They have 'Alzheimer's brains' but no symptoms. A new wave of drug developers wants to know why." STAT, February 27, 2020. https://www.statnews.com/2020/02/27/alzheimers-brains-but-no-symptoms/. Accesed April 29, 2021.

196. Davis M, T OC, Johnson S, et al. "Estimating Alzheimer's Disease Progression Rates from Normal Cognition Through Mild Cognitive Impairment and Stages of Dementia." *Curr Alzheimer Res.* 2018;15(8):777-788. doi:10.2174/1567205015666180119092427.

197. Lin Y, Shan PY, Jiang WJ, Sheng C, Ma L. "Subjective cognitive decline: preclinical manifestation of Alzheimer's disease." *Neurol Sci.* Jan 2019;40(1):41-49. doi:10.1007/s10072-018-3620-y.

198. Horgan D, Nobili F, Teunissen C, et al. "Biomarker Testing: Piercing the Fog of Alzheimer's and Related Dementia." *Biomed Hub.* Sep-Dec 2020;5(3):19-40. doi:10.1159/000511233.

199. Jack CR, Jr., Knopman DS, Jagust WJ, et al. "Tracking pathophysiological processes in Alzheimer's disease: an updated hypothetical model of dynamic biomarkers." *Lancet Neurol.* Feb 2013;12(2):207-16. doi:10.1016 /S1474-4422(12)70291-0.

200. Rossini PM, Di Iorio R, Vecchio F, et al. "Early diagnosis of Alzheimer's disease: the role of biomarkers including advanced EEG signal analysis. Report from the IFCN-sponsored panel of experts." *Clin Neurophysiol.* Jun 2020;131(6):1287-1310. doi:10.1016/j. clinph.2020.03.003.

201. Arnold SE. "'Senior Moments' or More? Diagnostic Evaluation of Cognitive Complaints in Older Adults and the Role of Cerebrospinal Fluid Biomarkers." *J Appl Lab Med.* Jan 1 2020;5(1):219-224. doi:10.1373 /jalm.2019.029546.

202. Ossenkoppele R, Smith R, Mattsson-Carlgren N, et al. "Accuracy of Tau Positron Emission Tomography as a Prognostic Marker in Preclinical and Prodromal Alzheimer Disease: A Head-to-Head Comparison Against Amyloid Positron Emission Tomography and Magnetic Resonance Imaging." *JAMA Neurol.* Jun 28 2021. doi:10.1001/jamaneurol.2021.1858.

203. Farid K, Caillat-Vigneron N, Sibon I. "Is brain SPECT useful in degenerative dementia diagnosis?" *J Comput Assist Tomogr.* Jan-Feb 2011;35(1):1-3. doi:10.1097 /RCT.0b013e3181f56fda.

204. Veitch DP, Weiner MW, Aisen PS, et al. "Understanding disease progression and improving Alzheimer's disease clinical trials: Recent highlights from the Alzheimer's Disease Neuroimaging Initiative." *Alzheimers Dement.* Jan 2019;15(1):106-152. doi:10.1016/j.jalz.2018.08.005.

205. Budson AE, Solomon PR. "Alzheimer's Disease." *Memory Loss, Alzheimer's Disease and Dementia.* 3 ed. Elsevier; 2022:49-72:chap 4.

206. Budson AE, Solomon PR. "Evaluating the Patient With Memory Loss or Dementia." *Memory Loss, Alzheimer's Disease and Dementia.* 3 ed. Elsevier; 2022:4-37:chap 2.

207. Piccirella S, Van Neste L, Fowler C, J. D, Uberti D, Kinnon P. "Alzosure® Predict, A Simple, Non-Invasive Blood Test To Predict The Early Onset Of Alzheimer's Disease With The Ability To Identify MCI Patients, Before The Clinical Symptoms Are Identifiable (In The Same Test) 6 Years In Advance Of Clinical Diagnosis." *J Prev Alzheimers Dis.* 2021;8(S1):s55-s56. doi:10.14283 /jpad.2021.57.

208. Liu J, Amin N, Arnold M, et al. "Profiling the metabolome of patients with dementia in the UK Biobank." *Alzheimer's & Dementia.* 2021;17(S5):e056147. doi:10.1002/alz.056147.

209. Cullen NC, Leuzy A, Janelidze S, et al. "Plasma biomarkers of Alzheimer's disease improve prediction of cognitive decline in cognitively unimpaired elderly populations." *Nat Commun.* Jun 11 2021;12(1):3555. doi:10.1038/s41467-021-23746-0.

210. Leuzy A, Cullen NC, Mattsson-Carlgren N, Hansson O. "Current advances in plasma and cerebrospinal fluid biomarkers in Alzheimer's disease." *Curr Opin Neurol.* Apr 1 2021;34(2):266-274. doi:10.1097 /WCO.0000000000000904.

211. Burke CW. "Blood Amyloid Test May Help Diagnose Alzheimer's, but Questions Remain." Alzforum. Dec 30 2022. https://www.alzforum.org/news/conference -coverage/blood-amyloid-test-may-help-diagnose- alzheimers-questions-remain. Accessed March 3, 2023.

212. Anderson J, Pierce C. "PrecivityAD for Diagnosis of Alzheimer Disease." *Am Fam Physician.* Jan 1 2022;105(1):79-81.

213. Schindler S. "First blood test for Alzheimer's disease." *AARP* magazine, October/November, 2021.

214. Schindler SE, Karikari TK, Ashton NJ, et al. "Effect of Race on Prediction of Brain Amyloidosis by Plasma Aβ42/Aβ40, Phosphorylated Tau, and Neurofilament Light." *Neurology.* Jul 19 2022;99(3):e245-e257. doi:10.1212/wnl.0000000000200358.

215. Galasko DR, Grill JD, Lingler JH, Heidebrink JL. "A Blood Test for Alzheimer's Disease: It's about Time or Not Ready for Prime Time?" *J Alzheimers Dis.* Feb 9 2022. doi:10.3233/jad-215490.

216. Pais MV, Forlenza OV, Diniz BS. "Plasma Biomarkers of Alzheimer's Disease: A Review of Available Assays, Recent Developments, and Implications for Clinical Practice." *J Alzheimers Dis Rep.* 2023;7(1):355-380. doi:10.3233/adr-230029.

217. Bahado-Singh RO, Vishweswaraiah S, Aydas B, et al. "Artificial intelligence and leukocyte epigenomics: Evaluation and prediction of late-onset Alzheimer's disease." *PLoS One.* 2021;16(3):e0248375. doi:10.1371/journal.pone.0248375.

218. Koychev I, Jansen K, Dette A, Shi L, Holling H. "Blood-Based ATN Biomarkers of Alzheimer's Disease: A Meta-Analysis." *J Alzheimers Dis.* 2021;79(1):177-195. doi:10.3233/JAD-200900.

219. Pacyna RR, Han SD, Wroblewski KE, McClintock MK, Pinto JM. "Rapid olfactory decline during aging predicts dementia and GMV loss in AD brain regions." *Alzheimers Dement.* Jul 28 2022. doi:10.1002/alz.12717.

220. Gonzalez-Aleman G. "Olfactory dysfunction but not COVID-19 severity predicts severity of cognitive

sequelae following SARS-CoV-2 infection in Amerindian older adults." The Alzheimer's Association International Conference (AAIC), Abstract 66868. Jul 31 2022. https://alz.confex.com/alz/2022 /meetingapp.cgi/Paper/66868.

221. Schindler S, Li Y, Buckles VD, et al. "Predicting Symptom Onset in Sporadic Alzheimer's Disease With Amyloid PET." *Neurology*. Sep 9 2021. doi:10.1212 /wnl.0000000000012775.

222. Koychev I, Vaci N, Bilgel M, et al. "Prediction of rapid amyloid and phosphorylated-Tau accumulation in cognitively healthy individuals." *Alzheimers Dement (Amst)*. 2020;12(1):e12019. doi:10.1002/dad2.12019.

223. Koychev I. "Medical focus must extend to pre-clinical dementia." YourLifeChoices, Apr 18 2021. https://www .yourlifechoices.com.au/health/medical-focus-must -extend-to-pre-clinical-dementia/. Accessed May 21, 2021.

224. Kapasi A, DeCarli C, Schneider JA. "Impact of multiple pathologies on the threshold for clinically overt dementia." *Acta Neuropathol*. Aug 2017;134(2):171-186. doi:10.1007/s00401-017-1717-7.

225. Visser PJ. "Use of biomarkers to select the target population for clinical trials in subjects with mild cognitive impairment." *The journal of nutrition, health & aging*. Apr 2009;13(4):344-5. doi:10.1007 /s12603-009-0037-6.

226. Dubois B, Villain N, Frisoni GB, et al. "Clinical diagnosis of Alzheimer's disease: recommendations of the International Working Group." *Lancet Neurol*. Jun 2021;20(6):484-496. doi:10.1016/s1474-4422 (21)00066-1.

227. 2022 "Alzheimer's disease facts and figures." *Alzheimers Dement*. Apr 2022;18(4):700-789. doi:10.1002/alz.12638.

228. Brookmeyer R, Abdalla N. "Estimation of lifetime risks of Alzheimer's disease dementia using biomarkers for preclinical disease." *Alzheimers Dement.* Aug 2018;14(8):981-988. doi:10.1016/j.jalz.2018.03.005.

229. Hemmy LS, Linskens EJ, Silverman PC, et al. "Brief Cognitive Tests for Distinguishing Clinical Alzheimer-Type Dementia From Mild Cognitive Impairment or Normal Cognition in Older Adults With Suspected Cognitive Impairment." *Ann Intern Med.* May 19 2020;172(10):678-687. doi:10.7326/m19-3889.

230. "Cognitive Tests Taken at Home Are on Par with In-Clinic Assessments." Alzforum. 2022. https://www .alzforum.org/news/conference-coverage/cognitive -tests-taken-home-are-par-clinic-assessments. Accessed January 2, 2023.

231. Budson AE, Solomon PR. "APPENDIX A: Cognitive Test and Questionnaire Forms, Instructions, and Normative Data for Evaluating Memory Loss, Alzheimer's Disease, and Dementia." *Memory Loss, Alzheimer's Disease and Dementia.* 3 ed. Elsevier; 2022:e1-e5.

232. Reardon CL. "Screening for Cognitive Impairment. Medscape." 2017. https://emedicine.medscape.com /article/1941498-overview. Accessed May 26, 2020.

233. Frellick M. "When to Refer Patients With New Memory Loss." Medscape. May 5 2021. https://www.medscape. com/viewarticle/950534. Accessed May 29, 2021.

234. Mendiondo MS, Ashford JW, Kryscio RJ, Schmitt FA. "Designing a Brief Alzheimer Screen (BAS)." *J Alzheimers Dis.* Oct 2003;5(5):391-8. doi:10.3233/jad-2003-5506.

235. O'Sullivan D, O'Regan NA, Timmons S. "Validity and Reliability of the 6-Item Cognitive Impairment Test for Screening Cognitive Impairment: A

Review." *Dement Geriatr Cogn Disord*. 2016;42(1-2):42-9. doi:10.1159/000448241.

236. Solomon PR, Hirschoff A, Kelly B, et al. "A 7-Minute Neurocognitive Screening Battery Highly Sensitive to Alzheimer's Disease." *Archives of Neurology*. 1998;55(3):349-355. doi:10.1001/archneur.55.3.349.

237. Szatloczki G, Hoffmann I, Vincze V, Kalman J, Pakaski M. "Speaking in Alzheimer's Disease, is That an Early Sign? Importance of Changes in Language Abilities in Alzheimer's Disease." *Front Aging Neurosci*. 2015;7:195. doi:10.3389/fnagi.2015.00195.

238. Mueller KD, Hermann B, Mecollari J, Turkstra LS. "Connected speech and language in mild cognitive impairment and Alzheimer's disease: A review of picture description tasks." *J Clin Exp Neuropsychol*. Nov 2018;40(9):917-939. doi:10.1080/13803395.2018.1446513.

239. Eyigoz E, Mathur S, Santamaria M, Cecchi G, Naylor M. "Linguistic markers predict onset of Alzheimer's disease." *EClinicalMedicine*. Nov 2020;28:100583. doi:10.1016/j.eclinm.2020.100583.

240. Kato S, Homma A, Sakuma T. "Easy Screening for Mild Alzheimer's Disease and Mild Cognitive Impairment from Elderly Speech." *Curr Alzheimer Res*. 2018;15(2):104-110. doi:10.2174/1567205014666171120144343.

241. Konig A, Satt A, Sorin A, et al. "Use of Speech Analyses within a Mobile Application for the Assessment of Cognitive Impairment in Elderly People." *Curr Alzheimer Res*. 2018;15(2):120-129. doi:10.2174/1567205014666170829111942.

242. Fraser KC, Meltzer JA, Rudzicz F. "Linguistic Features Identify Alzheimer's Disease in Narrative Speech." *J*

Alzheimers Dis. 2016;49(2):407-22. doi:10.3233/JAD-150520.

243. Mueller KD, Koscik RL, Hermann BP, Johnson SC, Turkstra LS. "Declines in Connected Language Are Associated with Very Early Mild Cognitive Impairment: Results from the Wisconsin Registry for Alzheimer's Prevention." *Front Aging Neurosci*. 2017;9:437. doi:10.3389/fnagi.2017.00437.

244. Mueller KD, Koscik RL, Turkstra LS, et al. "Connected Language in Late Middle-Aged Adults at Risk for Alzheimer's Disease." *J Alzheimers Dis*. Oct 18 2016;54(4):1539-1550. doi:10.3233/JAD-160252.

245. Sherman JC, Henderson CR, Jr., Flynn S, Gair JW, Lust B. "Language Decline Characterizes Amnestic Mild Cognitive Impairment Independent of Cognitive Decline." *J Speech Lang Hear Res*. Nov 8 2021;64(11):4287-4307. doi:10.1044/2021_jslhr-20-00503.

246. Berisha V, Wang S, LaCross A, Liss J. "Tracking discourse complexity preceding Alzheimer's disease diagnosis: a case study comparing the press conferences of Presidents Ronald Reagan and George Herbert Walker Bush." *J Alzheimers Dis*. 2015;45(3):959-63. doi:10.3233/jad-142763.

247. Bittner D, Frankenberg C, Schröder J. "Changes in Pronoun Use a Decade before Clinical Diagnosis of Alzheimer's Dementia-Linguistic Contexts Suggest Problems in Perspective-Taking." *Brain Sci*. Jan 17 2022;12(1). doi:10.3390/brainsci12010121.

248. Almor A, Kempler D, MacDonald MC, Andersen ES, Tyler LK. "Why do Alzheimer patients have difficulty with pronouns? Working memory, semantics, and reference in comprehension and production in

Alzheimer's disease." *Brain Lang.* May 1999;67(3):202-27. doi:10.1006/brln.1999.2055.

249. van Velzen MH, Nanetti L, de Deyn PP. "Data modelling in corpus linguistics: how low may we go?" *Cortex.* Jun 2014;55:192-201. doi:10.1016/j.cortex.2013.10.010.

250. Tran T. "Analysis of Language for Dementia Diagnosis with Focus on Alzheimer's Disease." 2017. https ://ttmt001.github.io/pdfs/ling575-proj2-report.pdf. Accessed May 26, 2020.

251. Lancashire E, Hirst G. "Vocabulary Changes in Agatha Christie's Mysteries as an Indication of Dementia: A Case Study." Presented at the 19th Annual Rotman Research Institute Conference, Cognitive Aging: Research and Practice, 8–10 March 2009, Toronto. https://www.researchgate.net/publication /242107161_Vocabulary_Changes_in _Agatha_Christie%27s_Mysteries_as_an_Indication _of_Dementia_A_Case_Study. Accessed July 5, 2020.

252. Delazer M, Zamarian L, Djamshidian A. "Handwriting in Alzheimer's Disease." *Journal of Alzheimer's Disease.* 2021;82:727-735. doi:10.3233/JAD-210279.

253. Saha R, Mukherjee A, Sadhukhan A, Roy A, De M. "Handwriting Analysis for Early Detection of Alzheimer's Disease." In: Gupta D, Bhattacharyya S, Khanna A, Sagar K, eds. *Intelligent Data Analysis: From Data Gathering to Data Comprehension.* Wiley; 2020:chap 18.

254. Souillard-Mandar W, Penney D, Schaible B, Pascual-Leone A, Au R, Davis R. "DCTclock: Clinically-Interpretable and Automated Artificial Intelligence Analysis of Drawing Behavior for Capturing Cognition." Original Research. *Frontiers in Digital Health.* Oct 15 2021;3doi:10.3389 /fdgth.2021.750661.

255. Rentz DM, Papp KV, Mayblyum DV, et al. "Association of Digital Clock Drawing With PET Amyloid and Tau Pathology in Normal Older Adults." *Neurology*. Apr 6 2021;96(14):e1844-e1854. doi:10.1212 /WNL.0000000000011697.

256. Kaido M, Fukui M, Kawashima M, Negishi K, Tsubota K. "Relationship between visual function and cognitive function in the elderly: A cross-sectional observational study." *PLoS One*. 2020;15(5):e0233381. doi:10.1371 /journal.pone.0233381.

257. McGrath R, Cawthon PM, Cesari M, Al Snih S, Clark BC. "Handgrip Strength Asymmetry and Weakness Are Associated with Lower Cognitive Function: A Panel Study." *J Am Geriatr Soc*. May 30 2020. doi:10.1111 /jgs.16556

258. Meysami S, Raji CA, Glatt RM, et al. "Handgrip Strength Is Related to Hippocampal and Lobar Brain Volumes in a Cohort of Cognitively Impaired Older Adults with Confirmed Amyloid Burden." *J Alzheimers Dis*. Dec 14 2022. doi:10.3233/JAD-220886.

259. Mirheidari B, Blackburn D, Harkness K, et al. "Toward the Automation of Diagnostic Conversation Analysis in Patients with Memory Complaints." *J Alzheimers Dis*. 2017;58(2):373-387. doi:10.3233/JAD-160507

260. Jarrold W, Peintner B, Wilkins DP, Richey C. "Aided Diagnosis of Dementia Type through Computer-Based Analysis of Spontaneous Speech." Conference Paper presented at Workshop on Computational Linguistics and Clinical Psychology: From Linguistic Signal to Clinical Reality, Baltimore, Maryland. June 27, 2014.

261. Zhou J, Lv Y, Mao C, et al. "Development and Validation of a Nomogram for Predicting the 6-Year Risk of Cognitive Impairment Among Chinese Older

Adults." *J Am Med Dir Assoc.* Jun 2020;21(6):864-871 e6. doi:10.1016/j.jamda.2020.03.032.

262. James C, Ranson JM, Everson R, Llewellyn DJ. "Performance of Machine Learning Algorithms for Predicting Progression to Dementia in Memory Clinic Patients." *JAMA Netw Open.* Dec 1 2021;4(12):e2136553. doi:10.1001/jamanetworkopen.2021.36553.

263. Brooks M. "FDA Clears 5-Minute Test doe Early Dementia." Medscape. Oct 20 2021. https://www .medscape.com/viewarticle/961277. Accessed October 31, 2021.

264. Liang X, Batsis JA, Zhu Y, et al. "Evaluating Voice-Assistant Commands for Dementia Detection." *Comput Speech Lang.* Mar 2022;72. doi:10.1016/j .csl.2021.101297.

265. Galvin JE, Roe CM, Powlishta KK, et al. "The AD8: a brief informant interview to detect dementia." *Neurology.* Aug 23 2005;65(4):559-64. doi:10.1212/01. wnl.0000172958.95282.2a.

266. Galvin JE, Roe CM, Coats MA, Morris JC. "Patient's rating of cognitive ability: using the AD8, a brief informant interview, as a self-rating tool to detect dementia." *Arch Neurol.* May 2007;64(5):725-30. doi:10.1001/archneur.64.5.725.

267. Chen HH, Sun FJ, Yeh TL, et al. "The diagnostic accuracy of the Ascertain Dementia 8 questionnaire for detecting cognitive impairment in primary care in the community, clinics and hospitals: a systematic review and meta-analysis." *Fam Pract.* May 23 2018;35(3):239-246. doi:10.1093/fampra/cmx098.

268. Frérot M, Lefebvre A, Aho S, Callier P, Astruc K, Aho Glélé LS. "What is epidemiology? Changing definitions of epidemiology 1978-2017." *PLoS*

One. 2018;13(12):e0208442. doi:10.1371/journal.
pone.0208442.

269. McCullough LE, Maliniak ML, Amin AB, et al.
"Epidemiology beyond its limits." *Sci Adv.* Jun 10
2022;8(23):eabn3328. doi:10.1126/sciadv.abn3328.

270. Stampfer MJ, Ridker PM, Dzau VJ. "Risk factor
criteria." *Circulation.* Jun 29 2004;109(25 Suppl 1):Iv3-5.
doi:10.1161/01.CIR.0000133446.69171.7d.

271. Cai H, Su N, Li W, Li X, Xiao S, Sun L. "Relationship
between afternoon napping and cognitive function
in the ageing Chinese population." *Gen Psychiatr.*
2021;34(1):e100361. doi:10.1136/gpsych-2020-100361.

272. Schneider AC, Moon C, Whitaker K, et al.
"Association of Sleep With Risk of Alzheimer's
Disease Mortality: NIH-AARP Diet and Health
Study." *J Appl Gerontol.* Apr 2022;41(4):1057-1065.
doi:10.1177/07334648211019207.

273. Li Y, Sahakian BJ, Kang J, et al. "The brain structure
and genetic mechanisms underlying the nonlinear
association between sleep duration, cognition and
mental health." *Nature Aging.* 2022/05/01 2022;2(5):425-
437. doi:10.1038/s43587-022-00210-2.

274. Ganguli M, Lee CW, Snitz BE, Hughes TF, McDade E,
Chang CC. "Rates and risk factors for progression to
incident dementia vary by age in a population cohort."
Neurology. Jan 6 2015;84(1):72-80. doi:10.1212
/WNL.0000000000001113.

275. Rahman A, Schelbaum E, Hoffman K, et al. "Sex-
driven modifiers of Alzheimer risk: A multimodality
brain imaging study." *Neurology.* Jun 24 2020. doi:10.1212
/WNL.0000000000009781.

276. Studart AN, Nitrini R. "Subjective cognitive decline:
The first clinical manifestation of Alzheimer's disease?"

Dement Neuropsychol. Jul-Sep 2016;10(3):170-177. doi:10.1590/S1980-5764-2016DN1003002.

277. Arboleda-Velasquez JF, Lopera F, O'Hare M, et al. "Resistance to autosomal dominant Alzheimer's disease in an APOE3 Christchurch homozygote: a case report." *Nat Med.* Nov 2019;25(11):1680-1683. doi:10.1038/s41591-019-0611-3.

278. Karlinsky H. "Alzheimer's disease in Down's syndrome. A review." *J Am Geriatr Soc.* Oct 1986;34(10):728-34. doi:10.1111/j.1532-5415.1986.tb04304.x.

279. Oliver C, Holland AJ. "Down's syndrome and Alzheimer's disease: a review." *Psychol Med.* May 1986;16(2):307-22. doi:10.1017/s0033291700009120.

280. Fortea J, Zaman SH, Hartley S, Rafii MS, Head E, Carmona-Iragui M. "Alzheimer's disease associated with Down syndrome: a genetic form of dementia." *Lancet Neurol.* Nov 2021;20(11):930-942. doi:10.1016/s1474-4422(21)00245-3.

281. Zhang B, Wang HE, Bai YM, et al. "Inflammatory bowel disease is associated with higher dementia risk: a nationwide longitudinal study." *Gut.* Jan 2021;70(1):85-91. doi:10.1136/gutjnl-2020-320789.

282. Zhang L, Du Rietz E, Kuja-Halkola R, et al. "Attention-deficit/hyperactivity disorder and Alzheimer's disease and any dementia: A multi-generation cohort study in Sweden." *Alzheimers Dement.* Sep 9 2021. doi:10.1002/alz.12462.

283. Bouzid H, Belk JA, Jan M, et al. "Clonal hematopoiesis is associated with protection from Alzheimer's disease." *Nat Med.* Jul 2023;29(7):1662-1670. doi:10.1038/s41591-023-02397-2.

284. Baumgart M, Snyder HM, Carrillo MC, Fazio S, Kim H, Johns H. "Summary of the evidence on modifiable

risk factors for cognitive decline and dementia: A population-based perspective." *Alzheimers Dement.* Jun 2015;11(6):718-26. doi:10.1016/j.jalz.2015.05.016.

285. National Institutes of Health, National Institute on Aging. "Cognitive Health and Older Adults." https ://www.nia.nih.gov/health/cognitive-health-and-older-adults. Accessed February 14, 2022.

286. Lee M, Whitsel E, Avery C, et al. "Variation in Population Attributable Fraction of Dementia Associated With Potentially Modifiable Risk Factors by Race and Ethnicity in the US." *JAMA Netw Open.* Jul 1 2022;5(7):e2219672. doi:10.1001 /jamanetworkopen.2022.19672.

287. Desai P, Evans D, Dhana K, et al. "Longitudinal Association of Total Tau Concentrations and Physical Activity With Cognitive Decline in a Population Sample." *JAMA Netw Open.* Aug 2 2021;4(8):e2120398. doi:10.1001/jamanetworkopen.2021.20398.

288. Brooks M. "Suicide Risk Jumps Soon After Dementia Diagnosis." Medscape. Aug 5 2021. https://www .medscape.com/viewarticle/956078. Accessed August 13, 2021.

289. Kivimaki M, Singh-Manoux A, Batty GD, et al. "Association of Alcohol-Induced Loss of Consciousness and Overall Alcohol Consumption With Risk for Dementia." *JAMA Netw Open.* Sep 1 2020;3(9):e2016084. doi:10.1001/jamanetworkopen.2020.16084.

290. Gomes Gonçalves N, Vidal Ferreira N, Khandpur N, et al. "Association Between Consumption of Ultraprocessed Foods and Cognitive Decline." *JAMA Neurol.* Dec 5 2022. doi:10.1001/jamaneurol.2022.4397.

291. Li H, Li S, Yang H, et al. "Association of Ultraprocessed Food Consumption With Risk of Dementia: A

Prospective Cohort." *Neurology*. Jul 27 2022. doi:10.1212/wnl.0000000000200871.

292. Meier MH, Caspi A, A RK, et al. "Long-Term Cannabis Use and Cognitive Reserves and Hippocampal Volume in Midlife." *Am J Psychiatry*. May 2022;179(5):362-374. doi:10.1176/appi.ajp.2021.21060664.

293. Winer JR, Deters KD, Kennedy G, et al. "Association of Short and Long Sleep Duration With Amyloid-β Burden and Cognition in Aging." *JAMA Neurol*. Aug 30 2021. doi:10.1001/jamaneurol.2021.2876

294. Li P, Gao L, Yu L, et al. "Daytime napping and Alzheimer's dementia: A potential bidirectional relationship." *Alzheimers Dement*. Mar 17 2022. doi:10.1002/alz.12636

295. de Menezes ST, Giatti L, Brant LCC, et al. "Hypertension, Prehypertension, and Hypertension Control: Association With Decline in Cognitive Performance in the ELSA-Brasil Cohort." *Hypertension*. Feb 2021;77(2):672-681. doi:10.1161/HYPERTENSIONAHA.120.16080.

296. Anderson P. "Antihypertensives Tied to Lower Alzheimer's Pathology." Medscape. Oct 25 2021. https://www.medscape.com/viewarticle/961531?ecd=ppc_google_rlsa-traf_mscp_news-perspectives_md-ldlm-cohort_us. Accessed November 16, 2021.

297. Peters R, Xu Y, Fitzgerald O, et al. "Blood pressure lowering and prevention of dementia: an individual patient data meta-analysis." *Eur Heart J*. Dec 21 2022;43(48):4980-4990. doi:10.1093/eurheartj/ehac584.

298. Mendez MF. "What is the Relationship of Traumatic Brain Injury to Dementia?" *J Alzheimers Dis*. 2017;57(3):667-681. doi:10.3233/JAD-161002.

299. Stevenson JS, Clifton L, Kuźma E, Littlejohns TJ. "Speech-in-noise hearing impairment is associated with an increased risk of incident dementia in 82,039 UK Biobank participants." *Alzheimers Dement.* Jul 21 2021;doi:10.1002/alz.12416.

300. Huang AR, Jiang K, Lin FR, Deal JA, Reed NS. "Hearing Loss and Dementia Prevalence in Older Adults in the US." *Jama.* Jan 10 2023;329(2):171-173. doi:10.1001/jama.2022.20954.

301. Bucholc M, McClean PL, Bauermeister S, et al. "Association of the use of hearing aids with the conversion from mild cognitive impairment to dementia and progression of dementia: A longitudinal retrospective study." *Alzheimers Dement.* 2021;7(1):e12122. doi:10.1002/trc2.12122

302. Bucholc M, Bauermeister S, Kaur D, McClean PL, Todd S. "The impact of hearing impairment and hearing aid use on progression to mild cognitive impairment in cognitively healthy adults: An observational cohort study." *Alzheimers Dement.* 2022;8(1):e12248. doi:10.1002/trc2.12248

303. Ehrlich JR, Goldstein J, Swenor BK, Whitson H, Langa KM, Veliz P. "Addition of Vision Impairment to a Life-Course Model of Potentially Modifiable Dementia Risk Factors in the US." *JAMA Neurol.* Jun 1 2022;79(6):623-626. doi:10.1001/jamaneurol.2022.0723.

304. Wang L, Davis PB, Volkow ND, Berger NA, Kaelber DC, Xu R. "Association of COVID-19 with New-Onset Alzheimer's Disease." *J Alzheimers Dis.* 2022;89(2):411-414. doi:10.3233/JAD-220717.

305. Cairns DM, Itzhaki RF, Kaplan DL. "Potential Involvement of Varicella Zoster Virus in Alzheimer's Disease via Reactivation of Quiescent Herpes Simplex

Virus Type 1." *J Alzheimers Dis.* 2022;88(3):1189-1200. doi:10.3233/jad-220287.

306. Rouch L, Vidal JS, Hoang T, Cestac P, Hanon O, Yaffe K. "Systolic blood pressure postural changes variability is associated with greater dementia risk." *Neurology.* Jul 20 2020. doi:10.1212/WNL.0000000000010420

307. Ehrenberg AJ, Suemoto CK, Franca Resende EP, et al. "Neuropathologic Correlates of Psychiatric Symptoms in Alzheimer's Disease." *J Alzheimers Dis.* 2018;66(1):115-126. doi:10.3233/JAD-180688

308. Anderson P. "Changes in Metabolism Tied to Risk of Subsequent Dementia." Medscape. Jul 28 2021. https://www.medscape.com/viewarticle/955575. Accessed December 3, 2021.

309. Otaiku AI. "Distressing dreams, cognitive decline, and risk of dementia: A prospective study of three population-based cohorts." eClinicalMedicine, Sep 21 2022. DOI:https://doi.org/10.1016/j.eclinm.2022.101640.

310. James B. "ICU hospitalization and incident dementia in community-based cohorts of older adults." The Alzheimer's Association International Conference (AAIC), Abstract 67719. Jul 31 2022.

311. Goldberg TE, Chen C, Wang Y, et al. "Association of Delirium With Long-term Cognitive Decline: A Meta-analysis." *JAMA Neurol.* Jul 13 2020. doi:10.1001/jamaneurol.2020.2273.

312. Cantuaria ML, Waldorff FB, Wermuth L, et al. "Residential exposure to transportation noise in Denmark and incidence of dementia: national cohort study." *BMJ.* Sep 8 2021;374:n1954. doi:10.1136/bmj.n1954.

313. Biddle KD, Jacobs HIL, d'Oleire Uquillas F, et al. "Associations of Widowhood and beta-Amyloid With

Cognitive Decline in Cognitively Unimpaired Older Adults." *JAMA Netw Open*. Feb 5 2020;3(2):e200121. doi:10.1001/jamanetworkopen.2020.0121.

314. Ngandu T, Lehtisalo J, Solomon A, et al. "A 2-year multidomain intervention of diet, exercise, cognitive training, and vascular risk monitoring versus control to prevent cognitive decline in at-risk elderly people (FINGER): a randomised controlled trial." *Lancet*. Jun 6 2015;385(9984):2255-63. doi:10.1016/s0140-6736(15)60461-5.

315. del Pozo Cruz B, Ahmadi M, Naismith SL, Stamatakis E. "Association of Daily Step Count and Intensity With Incident Dementia in 78, 430 Adults Living in the UK." *JAMA Neurology*. 2022;79(10):1059-1063. doi:10.1001/jamaneurol.2022.2672.

316. Yu JT, Xu W, Tan CC, et al. "Evidence-based prevention of Alzheimer's disease: systematic review and meta-analysis of 243 observational prospective studies and 153 randomised controlled trials." *J Neurol Neurosurg Psychiatry*. Jul 20 2020;doi:10.1136/jnnp-2019-321913.

317. Dhana K, Evans DA, Rajan KB, Bennett DA, Morris MC. "Healthy lifestyle and the risk of Alzheimer dementia: Findings from 2 longitudinal studies." *Neurology*. Jul 28 2020;95(4):e374-e383. doi:10.1212/WNL.0000000000009816.

318. Marchant NL, Lovland LR, Jones R, et al. "Repetitive negative thinking is associated with amyloid, tau, and cognitive decline." *Alzheimers Dement*. Jun 7 2020;doi:10.1002/alz.12116.

319. Hummel KV, Trautmann S, Venz J, Thomas S, Schafer J. "Repetitive negative thinking: transdiagnostic correlate and risk factor for mental disorders? A proof-of-concept study in German soldiers before and after

deployment to Afghanistan." *BMC Psychol.* Dec 19 2021;9(1):198. doi:10.1186/s40359-021-00696-2.

320. Nguyen HLT, Scambray KA, Sajjadi SA. Anti- "Hypertensive Medication Use is Associated with Decreased Likelihood of Neurodegenerative Pathologies." 146th Annual Meeting American Neurological Association. Abstract 375. Presented October 18, 2021. *Ann Neurol.* 2021;90(27):S86-S87.

321. Dhana K, James BD, Agarwal P, et al. "MIND Diet, Common Brain Pathologies, and Cognition in Community-Dwelling Older Adults." *J Alzheimers Dis.* 2021;83(2):683-692. doi:10.3233/jad-210107.

322. Zhang Y, Yang H, Li S, Li WD, Wang Y. "Consumption of coffee and tea and risk of developing stroke, dementia, and poststroke dementia: A cohort study in the UK Biobank." *PLoS medicine.* Nov 2021;18(11):e1003830. doi:10.1371/journal .pmed.1003830.

323. Zhang R, Shen L, Miles T, et al. "Association of Low to Moderate Alcohol Drinking With Cognitive Functions From Middle to Older Age Among US Adults." *JAMA Netw Open.* Jun 1 2020;3(6):e207922. doi:10.1001 /jamanetworkopen.2020.7922.

324. Jeon KH, Han K, Jeong SM, et al. "Changes in Alcohol Consumption and Risk of Dementia in a Nationwide Cohort in South Korea." *JAMA Netw Open.* Feb 1 2023;6(2):e2254771. doi:10.1001/ jamanetworkopen.2022.54771.

325. Fajersztajn L, Di Rienzo V, Nakamura CA, Scazufca M. "Watching TV and Cognition: The SPAH 2-Year Cohort Study of Older Adults Living in Low-Income Communities." *Front Neurol.* 2021;12:628489. doi:10.3389/fneur.2021.628489.

326. Fancourt D, Steptoe A. "Television viewing and cognitive decline in older age: findings from the English Longitudinal Study of Ageing." *Scientific Reports.* 2019/02/28 2019;9(1):2851. doi:10.1038 /s41598-019-39354-4.

327. Sabia S, Fayosse A, Dumurgier J, et al. "Association of sleep duration in middle and old age with incidence of dementia." *Nat Commun.* Apr 20 2021;12(1):2289. doi:10.1038/s41467-021-22354-2.

328. Ma Y, Liang L, Zheng F, Shi L, Zhong B, Xie W. "Association Between Sleep Duration and Cognitive Decline." *JAMA Netw Open.* Sep 1 2020;3(9):e2013573. doi:10.1001/jamanetworkopen.2020.13573.

329. Zhu Q, You Y, Fan L, Fan H. "Associations between sleep duration patterns and cognitive decline trajectories in older Chinese adults." *Aging Clin Exp Res.* Apr 10 2021;doi:10.1007/s40520-021-01851-w.

330. Lucey BP, Wisch J, Boerwinkle AH, et al. "Sleep and longitudinal cognitive performance in preclinical and early symptomatic Alzheimer's disease." *Brain.* Oct 20 2021;144(9):2852-62. doi:10.1093/brain/awab272.

331. McKee AC, Abdolmohammadi B, Stein TD. "The neuropathology of chronic traumatic encephalopathy." *Handb Clin Neurol.* 2018;158:297-307. doi:10.1016/ b978-0-444-63954-7.00028-8.

332. Nishimura K, Cordeiro JG, Ahmed AI, Yokobori S, Gajavelli S. "Advances in Traumatic Brain Injury Biomarkers." *Cureus.* Apr 2022;14(4):e23804. doi:10.7759/cureus.23804

333. Aiello Bowles EJ, Crane PK, Walker RL, et al. "Cognitive Resilience to Alzheimer's Disease Pathology in the Human Brain." *J Alzheimers Dis.* 2019;68(3):1071-1083. doi:10.3233/jad-180942.

334. Qiu C, Fratiglioni L. "Aging without Dementia is Achievable: Current Evidence from Epidemiological Research." *J Alzheimers Dis*. 2018;62(3):933-942. doi:10.3233/JAD-171037.

335. National Academies of Sciences, Engineering, and Medicine 2020. "Brain Health Across the Life Span: Proceedings of a Workshop." Washington, DC: The National Academies Press, 2020. https://doi .org/10.17226/25703.

336. Griciuc A, Serrano-Pozo A, Parrado AR, et al. "Alzheimer's disease risk gene CD33 inhibits microglial uptake of amyloid beta." *Neuron*. May 22 2013;78(4):631-43. doi:10.1016/j.neuron.2013.04.014.

337. Begley S. "She was destined to get early Alzheimer's, but didn't. Did a rare mutation protect her?" STAT. Nov 4 2019. https://www.statnews.com/2019/11/04/did -rare-mutation-protect-against-alzheimers/. Accessed April 13, 2022.

338. Lojo-Seoane C, Facal D, Guardia-Olmos J, Pereiro AX, Juncos-Rabadan O. "Effects of Cognitive Reserve on Cognitive Performance in a Follow-Up Study in Older Adults With Subjective Cognitive Complaints. The Role of Working Memory." *Front Aging Neurosci*. 2018;10:189. doi:10.3389/fnagi.2018.00189.

339. Pietzuch M, King AE, Ward DD, Vickers JC. "The Influence of Genetic Factors and Cognitive Reserve on Structural and Functional Resting-State Brain Networks in Aging and Alzheimer's Disease." *Front Aging Neurosci*. 2019;11:30. doi:10.3389/fnagi.2019.00030.

340. Rentz DM, Locascio JJ, Becker JA, et al. "Cognition, reserve, and amyloid deposition in normal aging." *Ann Neurol*. Mar 2010;67(3):353-64. doi:10.1002/ana.21904.

341. Fischer FU, Wolf D, Tuscher O, Fellgiebel A, "Alzheimer's Disease Neuroimaging I. Structural Network Efficiency Predicts Resilience to Cognitive Decline in Elderly at Risk for Alzheimer's Disease." *Front Aging Neurosci.* 2021;13:637002. doi:10.3389 /fnagi.2021.637002.

342. Kivimaki M, Walker KA, Pentti J, et al. "Cognitive stimulation in the workplace, plasma proteins, and risk of dementia: three analyses of population cohort studies." *BMJ.* Aug 18 2021;374:n1804. doi:10.1136 /bmj.n1804.

343. Oveisgharan S, Wilson RS, Yu L, Schneider JA, Bennett DA. "Association of Early-Life Cognitive Enrichment With Alzheimer Disease Pathological Changes and Cognitive Decline." *JAMA Neurol.* Jun 29 2020;doi:10.1001/jamaneurol.2020.1941.

344. Hohman TJ, Kaczorowski CC. "Modifiable Lifestyle Factors in Alzheimer Disease: An Opportunity to Transform the Therapeutic Landscape Through Transdisciplinary Collaboration." *JAMA Neurol.* Jun 29 2020;doi:10.1001/jamaneurol.2020.1114.

345. McMaster M, Kim S, Clare L, Torres SJ, D'Este C, Anstey KJ. "Body, Brain, Life for Cognitive Decline (BBL-CD): protocol for a multidomain dementia risk reduction randomized controlled trial for subjective cognitive decline and mild cognitive impairment." *Clin Interv Aging.* 2018;13:2397-2406. doi:10.2147/CIA. S182046.

346. McMaster M, Kim S, Clare L, et al. "Lifestyle Risk Factors and Cognitive Outcomes from the Multidomain Dementia Risk Reduction Randomized Controlled Trial, Body Brain Life for Cognitive Decline

(BBL-CD)." *J Am Geriatr Soc*. Nov 2020;68(11):2629-2637. doi:10.1111/jgs.16762.

347. Jeong SH, Kim HR, Kim J, et al. "Association of Dipeptidyl Peptidase-4 Inhibitor Use and Amyloid Burden in Diabetic Patients With AD-Related Cognitive Impairment." *Neurology*. Aug 11 2021;doi:10.1212/WNL.0000000000012534.

348. McKeith IG, Boeve BF, Dickson DW, et al. "Diagnosis and management of dementia with Lewy bodies: Fourth consensus report of the DLB Consortium." *Neurology*. Jul 4 2017;89(1):88-100. doi:10.1212/wnl.0000000000004058.

349. Reed J. "Dementia with a Difference: Exploring Causes of Frontotemporal Dementia—and Potential Treatments." *Brain&Life*, April/May 2021, pp.32-35. The American Academy of Neurology. https://www.brainandlife.org/disorders-a-z/disorders/alzheimer-s-disease/organizations. Accessed June 6, 2021.

350. Puppala GK, Gorthi SP, Chandran V, Gundabolu G. "Frontotemporal Dementia—Current Concepts." *Neurol India*. Sep-Oct 2021;69(5):1144-1152. doi:10.4103/0028-3886.329593.

351. Nelson PT, Dickson DW, Trojanowski JQ, et al. "Limbic-predominant age-related TDP-43 encephalopathy (LATE): consensus working group report." *Brain*. Jun 1 2019;142(6):1503-1527. doi:10.1093/brain/awz099.

352. Duong MT, Wolk DA. "Limbic-Predominant Age-Related TDP-43 Encephalopathy: LATE-Breaking Updates in Clinicopathologic Features and Biomarkers." *Curr Neurol Neurosci Rep*. Nov 2022;22(11):689-698. doi:10.1007/s11910-022-01232-4.

353. Nelson PT, Schneider JA, Jicha GA, Duong MT, Wolk DA. "When Alzheimer's is LATE: Why Does it Matter?"

Ann Neurol. Aug 2023;94(2):211-222. doi:10.1002 /ana.26711.

354. Townley RA, Graff-Radford J, Mantyh WG, et al. "Progressive dysexecutive syndrome due to Alzheimer's disease: a description of 55 cases and comparison to other phenotypes." *Brain Commun.* 2020;2(1):fcaa068. doi:10.1093/braincomms/fcaa068.

355. Hellmuth J, Barnett TA, Asken BM, et al. "Persistent COVID-19-associated neurocognitive symptoms in non-hospitalized patients." *J Neurovirol.* Feb 2021;27(1): 191-195. doi:10.1007/s13365-021-00954-4.

356. Salamanna F, Veronesi F, Martini L, Landini MP, Fini M. "Post-COVID-19 Syndrome: The Persistent Symptoms at the Post-viral Stage of the Disease. A Systematic Review of the Current Data." *Front Med (Lausanne).* 2021;8:653516. doi:10.3389 /fmed.2021.653516.

357. Graham EL, Clark JR, Orban ZS, et al. "Persistent neurologic symptoms and cognitive dysfunction in non-hospitalized Covid-19 'long haulers.'" *Ann Clin Transl Neurol.* May 2021;8(5):1073-1085. doi:10.1002 /acn3.51350.

358. Chatterjee R. "If Your Brain Feels Foggy And You're Tired All The Time, You're Not Alone." National Public Radio, May 7, 2021. https://www.npr.org/sections /health-shots/2021/05/06/992401123/if-your-brain -feels-foggy-and-youre-tired-all-the-time-youre-not -alone. Accessed June 14, 2021.

359. Vacas S, Cole DJ, Cannesson M. "Cognitive Decline Associated With Anesthesia and Surgery in Older Patients." *JAMA.* Aug 2 2021;doi:10.1001 /jama.2021.4773. https://jamanetwork.com/journals /jama/fullarticle/2782851 Accessed August 13, 2021.

360. Budson AE, Solomon PR. "Other Disorders That Cause Memory Loss or Dementia." *Memory Loss, Alzheimer's Disease and Dementia*. 3 ed. Elsevier; 2022:186-197:chap 17.

361. Barrett AM. "Is it Alzheimer's disease or something else? 10 disorders that may feature impaired memory and cognition." *Postgrad Med*. May 2005;117(5):47-53.

362. Taragano FE, Allegri RF, Heisecke SL, et al. "Risk of Conversion to Dementia in a Mild Behavioral Impairment Group Compared to a Psychiatric Group and to a Mild Cognitive Impairment Group." *J Alzheimers Dis*. 2018;62(1):227-238. doi:10.3233/JAD-170632.

363. Taragano FE, Allegri RF, Lyketsos C. "Mild behavioral impairment: A prodromal stage of dementia." *Dement Neuropsychol*. Oct-Dec 2008;2(4):256-260. doi:10.1590/S1980-57642009DN20400004.

364. Creese B, Ismail Z. "Mild behavioral impairment: measurement and clinical correlates of a novel marker of preclinical Alzheimer's disease." *Alzheimers Res Ther*. Jan 5 2022;14(1):2. doi:10.1186/s13195-021-00949-7.

365. Taragano FE, Allegri RF, Krupitzki H, et al. "Mild behavioral impairment and risk of dementia: a prospective cohort study of 358 patients." *J Clin Psychiatry*. Apr 2009;70(4):584-92. doi:10.4088/jcp.08m04181.

366. Swaddiwudhipong N, Whiteside DJ, Hezemans FH, Street D, Rowe JB, Rittman T. "Pre-diagnostic cognitive and functional impairment in multiple sporadic neurodegenerative diseases." *Alzheimers Dement*. Oct 12 2022;doi:10.1002/alz.12802.

367. Haaksma ML, Eriksdotter M, Rizzuto D, et al. "Survival time tool to guide care planning in people with dementia." *Neurology*. 2020;94(5):e538-e548. doi:10.1212/wnl.0000000000008745

368. Sampson EL. "Palliative care for people with dementia." *Br Med Bull.* 2010;96:159-74. doi:10.1093/bmb/ldq024.

369. "Guiding principles for the care of older adults with multimorbidity: an approach for clinicians: American Geriatrics Society Expert Panel on the Care of Older Adults with Multimorbidity." *J Am Geriatr Soc.* Oct 2012;60(10):E1-e25. doi:10.1111/j.1532-5415.2012.04188.x.

370. Alothman D, Card T, Lewis S, Tyrrell E, Fogarty AW, Marshall CR. "Risk of Suicide After Dementia Diagnosis." *JAMA Neurol.* Oct 3 2022;79(11):1148-54. doi:10.1001/jamaneurol.2022.3094.

371. Choi JW, Lee KS, Han E. "Suicide risk within 1 year of dementia diagnosis in older adults: a nationwide retrospective cohort study." *J Psychiatry Neurosci.* Jan 4 2021;46(1):E119-e127. doi:10.1503/jpn.190219.

372. Lee YF, Hsu TW, Liang CS, et al. "The Efficacy and Safety of Tube Feeding in Advanced Dementia Patients: A Systemic Review and Meta-Analysis Study." *J Am Med Dir Assoc.* Feb 2021;22(2):357-363. doi:10.1016/j.jamda.2020.06.035.

373. Sampson EL, Candy B, Jones L. "Enteral tube feeding for older people with advanced dementia." *Cochrane Database Syst Rev.* Apr 15 2009;2009(2):Cd007209. doi:10.1002/14651858.CD007209.pub2.

374. Budson AE, Solomon PR. "Life Adjustments for Memory Loss, Alzheimer's Disease, and Dementia." *Memory Loss, Alzheimer's Disease and Dementia.* 3 ed. Elsevier; 2022:287-292:chap 28.

375. In: Larson EB, Stroud C, eds. *Meeting the Challenge of Caring for Persons Living with Dementia and Their Care Partners and Caregivers: A Way Forward.* 2021. The National

Academies Collection: Reports funded by National
Institutes of Health.

376. Budson AE, Solomon PR. "Caring for and Educating
the Caregiver." *Memory Loss, Alzheimer's Disease and
Dementia*. 3 ed. Elsevier; 2022:261-266:chap 25.

377. Gitlin L, Jutkowitz E, Gaugler JE. Dementia Caregiver
Intervention Research Now and into the Future: Review
and Recommendations. Paper prepared for the National
Academies of Sciences, Engineering, and Medicine,
Decadal Survey of Behavioral and Social Science
Research on Alzheimer's Disease and Alzheimer's
Disease-Related Dementias. https://sites
.nationalacademies.org/cs/groups/dbassesite
/documents/webpage/dbasse_198208.pdf. Accesed
June 22, 2022.

378. Butler M, Gaugler JE, Talley KMC, et al. *Care
Interventions for People Living With Dementia and Their
Caregivers. Comparative Effectiveness Review No. 231.*
(Prepared by the Minnesota Evidence-based Practice
Center under Contract No. 290-2015-00008-I.) AHRQ
Publication No. 20-EHC023. Rockville, MD: Agency
for Healthcare Research and Quality; August 2020.
https://effectivehealthcare.ahrq.gov/sites/default/files
/cer-231-dementia-interventions-evidence-summary_0.
pdf. Accessed June 22, 2022.

379. Choi H, Heisler M, Norton EC, Langa KM, Cho TC,
Connell CM. "Family Care Availability And Implications
For Informal And Formal Care Used By Adults With
Dementia In The US." *Health Aff (Millwood)*. Sep
2021;40(9):1359-1367. doi:10.1377/hlthaff.2021.00280.

380. McFarlane R, Bashe P. *The complete bedside companion
: no-nonsense advice on caring for the seriously ill*. Simon &
Schuster; 1998.

381. Budson AE, K. O'Connor M. *Six steps to managing Alzheimer's disease and Dementia : a guide for families*. Oxford University Press; 2021.

382. Mace NL, Rabins PV. *The 36-hour day : a family guide to caring for people who have Alzheimer disease, other dementias, and memory loss*. 6th edition. ed. Johns Hopkins University Press; 2017:xx.

383. Prince M, Comas-Herrera A, Knapp M, Guerchet M, Karagiannidou M. "World Alzheimer report 2016: improving healthcare for people living with dementia: coverage, quality and costs now and in the future." Alzheimer's Disease International (ADI), London, UK. http://eprints.lse.ac.uk/67858/1/Comas-Herrera _World%20Alzheimer%20report_2016.pdf. Accessed August 2, 2020.

384. National Academies of Sciences E, Medicine, Division of B, et al. The National Academies Collection: Reports funded by National Institutes of Health. *Understanding Nursing Home, Hospice, and Palliative Care for Individuals with Later-Stage Dementia: Proceedings of a Workshop—in Brief*. National Academies Press (US), 2020.

385. Wynn P. "Expert Advice for Finding the Right Home Health Aide." *Brain&Life*, June/July, 2021. https://www .brainandlife.org/articles/expert-advice-finding-home -health-aide/. Accessed August 13, 2021.

386. Budson AE, Solomon PR. "Legal and Financial Issues in Memory Loss, Alzheimer's Disease, and Dementia." *Memory Loss, Alzheimer's Disease and Dementia*. 3 ed. Elsevier; 2022:293-296:chap 29.

387. Etchells E, Sharpe G, Elliott C, Singer PA. "Bioethics for clinicians: 3. Capacity." *Cmaj*. Sep 15 1996;155(6):657-61.

388. Patnode CD, Perdue LA, Rossom RC, et al. U.S. Preventive Services Task Force Evidence Syntheses, formerly Systematic Evidence Reviews. *Screening for*

Cognitive Impairment in Older Adults: An Evidence Update for the US Preventive Services Task Force. Agency for Healthcare Research and Quality (US); 2020.

389. Patnode CD, Perdue LA, Rossom RC, et al. "Screening for Cognitive Impairment in Older Adults: Updated Evidence Report and Systematic Review for the US Preventive Services Task Force." *JAMA*. Feb 25 2020;323(8):764-785. doi:10.1001/jama.2019.22258.

390. Revi M. "Alzheimer's Disease Therapeutic Approaches." *Adv Exp Med Biol*. 2020;1195:105-116. doi:10.1007/978-3-030-32633-3_15.

391. Cummings J, Lee G, Ritter A, Sabbagh M, Zhong K. "Alzheimer's disease drug development pipeline: 2019." *Alzheimers Dement*. 2019;5:272-293. doi:10.1016/j .trci.2019.05.008.

392. Cummings J, Lee G, Nahed P, et al. "Alzheimer's disease drug development pipeline: 2022." *Alzheimers Dement*. 2022;8(1):e12295. doi:10.1002/trc2.12295.

393. Sperling RA, Jack CR, Jr., Aisen PS. "Testing the right target and right drug at the right stage." *Sci Transl Med*. Nov 30 2011;3(111):111cm33. doi:10.1126 /scitranslmed.3002609.

394. Gunter J. "The Truth About Our Bodies." NPR. May 28, 2021. https://www.npr.org/transcripts/1000902810. Accessed May 3, 2023.

395. Budson AE, Solomon PR. "Why Diagnose and Treat Memory Loss, Alzheimer's Disease, and Dementia?" *Memory Loss, Alzheimer's Disease and Dementia*. 3 ed. Elsevier; 2022:1-3:chap 1.

396. Hao Y, Dong M, Sun Y, Duan X, Niu W. "Effectiveness and safety of monoclonal antibodies against amyloid-beta vis-à-vis placebo in mild or moderate Alzheimer's disease." *Front Neurol*. 2023;14:1147757. doi:10.3389 /fneur.2023.1147757.

397. Lacorte E, Ancidoni A, Zaccaria V, et al. Safety and "Efficacy of Monoclonal Antibodies for Alzheimer's Disease: A Systematic Review and Meta-Analysis of Published and Unpublished Clinical Trials." *J Alzheimers Dis.* 2022;87(1):101-129. doi:10.3233/JAD-220046.

398. Tampi RR, Forester BP, Agronin M. "Aducanumab: evidence from clinical trial data and controversies." *Drugs Context.* 2021;10. doi:10.7573/dic.2021-7-3.

399. Robinson JC. "Why Is Aducanumab Priced at $56,000 per Patient? Lessons for Drug-Pricing Reform." *N Engl J Med.* Nov 25 2021;385(22):2017-2019. doi:10.1056/NEJMp2113679.

400. Alexander GC, Emerson S, Kesselheim AS. "Evaluation of Aducanumab for Alzheimer Disease: Scientific Evidence and Regulatory Review Involving Efficacy, Safety, and Futility." *JAMA.* Mar 30 2021;doi:10.1001/jama.2021.3854.

401. Chiong W, Tolchin BD, Bonnie RJ, et al. "Decisions With Patients and Families Regarding Aducanumab in Alzheimer Disease, With Recommendations for Consent: AAN Position Statement." *Neurology.* Nov 17 2021;doi:10.1212/wnl.0000000000013053.

402. Salloway S, Chalkias S, Barkhof F, et al. "Amyloid -Related Imaging Abnormalities in 2 Phase 3 Studies Evaluating Aducanumab in Patients With Early Alzheimer Disease." *JAMA Neurol.* Nov 22 2021;doi:10.1001/jamaneurol.2021.4161.

403. Belluck P. "Treating Alzheimer's Very Early Offers Better Hope of Slowing Decline, Study Finds." *New York Times,* July 17, 2023. https://www.nytimes.com/2023/07/17/health/alzheimers-drug-donanemab.html. Accessed August 5, 2023; Belluck P. "Cleveland Clinic and Mount Sinai Won't Administer Aduhelm to Patients." *New York Times,* July 14, 2021. https://www.nytimes

.com/2021/07/14/health/cleveland-clinic-aduhelm
.html. Accessed July 22, 2021.

404. Alzheimer's Association. "Alzheimer's Association
Statement on CMS Draft Decision." January 11, 2022.
https://www.google.com/url?sa=t&rct=j&q=&esrc=s
&source=web&cd=&ved=2ahUKEwjB8-zI3vz1AhUKl
YkEHSiGC44QFnoECAIQAQ&url=https%3A%2F%
2Fwww.alz.org%2Fnews%2F2022%2Falzheimers
-association-statement-on-cms-draft-deci&usg=AOvVaw
2fafry325q0qdF8qqGCGNa; www.alz.org/news/2022
/alzheimers-association-statement-on-cms-draft-deci.
Accessed February 13, 2022.

405. Karlawish J. "Aducanumab and the Business of
Alzheimer Disease—Some Choice." *JAMA Neurol.* Aug
19 2021;doi:10.1001/jamaneurol.2021.3123.

406. van Dyck CH, Swanson CJ, Aisen P, et al. "Lecanemab
in Early Alzheimer's Disease." *N Engl J Med.* Jan 5
2023;388(1):9-21. doi:10.1056/NEJMoa2212948.

407. Qiao Y, Chi Y, Zhang Q, Ma Y. "Safety and efficacy of
lecanemab for Alzheimer's disease: a systematic review
and meta-analysis of randomized clinical trials." *Front
Aging Neurosci.* 2023;15:1169499. doi:10.3389
/fnagi.2023.1169499.

408. Lansdall CJ, McDougall F, Butler LM, et al.
"Establishing Clinically Meaningful Change on
Outcome Assessments Frequently Used in Trials of Mild
Cognitive Impairment Due to Alzheimer's Disease."
J Prev Alzheimers Dis. 2023;10(1):9-18. doi:10.14283
/jpad.2022.102.

409. Hendrix SB, Dickson SP. "Editorial: Usefulness of
Anchor-Based Methods for Determining Clinically
Meaningful Change in MCI due to AD." *J Prev Alzheimers
Dis.* 2023;10(1):7-8. doi:10.14283/jpad.2022.104.

410. Rogers MB. "Donanemab Mops Up Plaque Faster Than Aduhelm." Alzforum. Dec 16 2022. https://www .alzforum.org/news/conference-coverage/donanemab -mops-plaque-faster-aduhelm#:~:text=As%20 expected%20based%20on%20earlier,first%20six%20 months%20of%20treatment. Accessed February 23, 2023.

411. Travis J. "Latest Alzheimer's antibody is 'not a miracle drug.'" *Science*. May 12 2023;380(6645):571. doi:10.1126 /science.adi6515.

412. Sims JR, Zimmer JA, Evans CD, et al. "Donanemab in Early Symptomatic Alzheimer Disease: The TRAILBLAZER-ALZ 2 Randomized Clinical Trial." *JAMA*. Jul 17 2023;doi:10.1001/jama.2023.13239.

413. "Lilly's Donanemab Significantly Slowed Cognitive and Functional Decline in Phase 3 Study of Early Alzheimer's Disease." [Press Release] May 3, 2023. https://www.prnewswire.com/news-releases /lillys-donanemab-significantly-slowed-cognitive-and -functional-decline-in-phase-3-study-of-early -alzheimers-disease-301814001.html.

414. Espay AJ. "Donanemab in Early Alzheimer's Disease." *N Engl J Med*. Aug 12 2021;385(7):666-667. doi:10.1056 /NEJMc2109455.

415. Wessels AM, Dennehy EB, Dowsett SA, Dickson SP, Hendrix SB. "Meaningful Clinical Changes in Alzheimer Disease Measured With the iADRS and Illustrated Using the Donanemab TRAILBLAZER-ALZ Study Findings." *Neurol Clin Pract*. Apr 2023;13(2):e200127. doi:10.1212/ cpj.0000000000200127.

416. Joseph-Mathurin N, Wang G, Kantarci K, et al. "Longitudinal Accumulation of Cerebral Microhemorrhages in Dominantly Inherited Alzheimer

Disease." *Neurology*. Mar 23 2021;96(12):e1632-e1645. doi:10.1212/WNL.0000000000011542.

417. Planche V, Villain N. "US Food and Drug Administration Approval of Aducanumab—Is Amyloid Load a Valid Surrogate End Point for Alzheimer Disease Clinical Trials?" *JAMA Neurology*. 2021;78(11):1307-1308. doi:10.1001/jamaneurol.2021.3126.

418. Ackley SF, Zimmerman SC, Brenowitz WD, et al. "Effect of reductions in amyloid levels on cognitive change in randomized trials: instrumental variable meta-analysis." *BMJ*. Feb 25 2021;372:n156. doi:10.1136/bmj.n156.

419. Doggrell SA. "Still grasping at straws: donanemab in Alzheimer's disease." *Expert Opin Investig Drugs*. Aug 2021;30(8):797-801. doi:10.1080/13543784.2021.1948010.

420. Karlawish J. "The FDA needs a risk evaluation and mitigation strategy for Alzheimer's drug lecanemab." STATNews.com. June 16, 2023. https://www.statnews.com/2023/06/16/the-fda-needs-a-risk-evaluation-and-mitigation-strategy-for-alzheimers-drug-lecanemab/Accessed August 4, 2023.

421. Cummings J. "Anti-Amyloid Monoclonal Antibodies are Transformative Treatments that Redefine Alzheimer's Disease Therapeutics." *Drugs*. May 2023;83(7):569-576. doi:10.1007/s40265-023-01858-9.

422. Doggrell SA. "Still grasping at straws: donanemab in Alzheimer's disease." *Expert Opin Investig Drugs*. Aug 2021;30(8):797-801. doi:10.1080/13543784.2021.1948010.

423. Widera EW, Brangman SA, Chin NA. "Ushering in a New Era of Alzheimer Disease Therapy." *JAMA*. 2023;doi:10.1001/jama.2023.11701.

424. Grodstein F, Leurgans SE, Capuano AW, Schneider JA, Bennett DA. "Trends in Postmortem Neurodegenerative

and Cerebrovascular Neuropathologies Over 25 Years."
JAMA Neurology. 2023;80(4):370-376. doi:10.1001
/jamaneurol.2022.5416.

425. Budson AE, Solomon PR. "Cholinesterase Inhibitors."
Memory Loss, Alzheimer's Disease and Dementia. 3 ed.
Elsevier; 2022:202-216:chap 19.

426. Budson AE, Solomon PR. "Memantine." *Memory Loss,
Alzheimer's Disease and Dementia.* 3 ed. Elsevier; 2022: 217-
223:chap 20.

427. Budson AE, Solomon PR. "Nonpharmacological
Treatment of Memory Loss, Alzheimer's Disease, and
Dementia." *Memory Loss, Alzheimer's Disease and Dementia.*
3 ed. Elsevier; 2022:231-236:chap 22.

428. Budson AE, Solomon, PR. "Nonpharmacological
Treatment of the Behavioral and Psychological
Symptoms of Dementia." *Memory Loss, Alzheimer's Disease
and Dementia.* 3 ed. Elsevier; 2022:267-275:chap 26.

429. "Brexpiprazole Eases Agitation in People with AD; So
Does Being in a Trial." Alzforum. 2022. https
://www.alzforum.org/news/conference-coverage
/brexpiprazole-eases-agitation-people-ad-so-does-being
-trial. Accessed January 2, 2023. https://www.alzforum
.org/news/conference-coverage/cognitive-tests-taken
-home-are-par-clinic-assessments. Accessed January 2,
2023.

430. Banerjee S, High J, Stirling S, et al. "Study of
mirtazapine for agitated behaviours in dementia
(SYMBAD): a randomised, double-blind, placebo-
controlled trial." *Lancet.* Oct 23 2021;398(10310):1487-
1497. doi:10.1016/s0140-6736(21)01210-1.

431. Parmer N. "The Rise of Dementia Villages—the
Happiest Places on Earth?" https://www.ozy.com/the
-new-and-the-next/the-rise-of-dementia-villages-the

-happiest-places-on-earth/79270/. Accessed October 13, 2022.

432. Budson AE, Solomon PR. "Goals for the Treatment of Memory Loss, Alzheimer's Disease, and Dementia." *Memory Loss, Alzheimer's Disease and Dementia*. 3 ed. Elsevier; 2022:199-201:chap 18.

433. Unverzagt FW, Guey LT, Jones RN, et al. "ACTIVE cognitive training and rates of incident dementia." *Journal of the International Neuropsychological Society: JINS*. Jul 2012;18(4):669-77. doi:10.1017/S13556177 11001470.

434. Rebok GW, Ball K, Guey LT, et al. "Ten-year effects of the advanced cognitive training for independent and vital elderly cognitive training trial on cognition and everyday functioning in older adults." *J Am Geriatr Soc*. Jan 2014;62(1):16-24. doi:10.1111/jgs.12607.

435. Jaeggi SM, Buschkuehl M, Jonides J, Perrig WJ. "Improving fluid intelligence with training on working memory." *Proc Natl Acad Sci U S A*. May 13 2008;105(19):6829-33. doi:10.1073/pnas.0801268105.

436. National Academies of Sciences, Engineering, and Medicine. *Preventing cognitive decline and dementia: a way forward*. The National Academies Press, 2017.

437. Budson AE, Solomon PR. "Vitamins, Herbs, Supplements, and Antiinflammatories." *Memory Loss, Alzheimer's Disease and Dementia*. 3 ed. Elsevier; 2022:224-230:chap 21.

438. Baker L, Manson J, Rapp S, et al. "Impact of Cocoa Flavanols and Multivitamins on Cognitive Function: Findings of the Cocoa Supplement and Multivitamin Outcomes Study of Cognition(COSMOS-MIND)." 14th Clinical Trials on Alzheimer's Disease (CTAD) conference: Oral communication (OC-11).

Presented November 10, 2021. *J Prev Alzheimers Dis.* 2021;8(S1):S19-s20. doi:10.14283/jpad.2021.57.

439. Yeung LK, Alschuler DM, Wall M, et al. "Multivitamin Supplementation Improves Memory in Older Adults: A Randomized Clinical Trial." *Am J Clin Nutr.* Jul 2023;118(1):273-282. doi:10.1016/j.ajcnut.2023.05.011.

440. Beydoun MA, Beydoun HA, Fanelli-Kuczmarski MT, et al. "Association of Serum Antioxidant Vitamins and Carotenoids With Incident Alzheimer Disease and All-Cause Dementia Among US Adults." *Neurology.* May 4 2022;doi:10.1212/wnl.0000000000200289.

441. Voulgaropoulou SD, van Amelsvoort T, Prickaerts J, Vingerhoets C. "The effect of curcumin on cognition in Alzheimer's disease and healthy aging: A systematic review of pre-clinical and clinical studies." *Brain Res.* Dec 15 2019;1725:146476. doi:10.1016/j .brainres.2019.146476.

442. Benameur T, Giacomucci G, Panaro MA, et al. "New Promising Therapeutic Avenues of Curcumin in Brain Diseases." *Molecules.* Dec 31 2021;27(1). doi:10.3390 /molecules27010236.

443. Tsai IC, Hsu CW, Chang CH, Tseng PT, Chang KV. "The Effect of Curcumin Differs on Individual Cognitive Domains across Different Patient Populations: A Systematic Review and Meta-Analysis." *Pharmaceuticals (Basel).* Nov 28 2021;14(12). doi:10.3390/ph14121235.

444. Gratton G, Weaver SR, Burley CV, et al. "Dietary flavanols improve cerebral cortical oxygenation and cognition in healthy adults." *Sci Rep.* Nov 24 2020;10(1):19409. doi:10.1038/s41598-020-76160-9.

445. Brickman AM, Khan UA, Provenzano FA, et al. "Enhancing dentate gyrus function with dietary flavanols improves cognition in older adults." *Nat Neurosci.* Dec 2014;17(12):1798-803. doi:10.1038/nn.3850.

446. Pa J, Gazzaley A. "Flavanol-rich food for thought." *Nat Neurosci*. Dec 2014;17(12):1624-5. doi:10.1038/nn.3876.

447. Flanagan E, Cameron D, Sobhan R, et al. "Chronic Consumption of Cranberries (Vaccinium macrocarpon) for 12 Weeks Improves Episodic Memory and Regional Brain Perfusion in Healthy Older Adults: A Randomised, Placebo-Controlled, Parallel-Groups Feasibility Study." Original Research. *Frontiers in Nutrition*. 2022-May-19 2022;9doi:10.3389/fnut.2022.849902.

448. Shishtar E, Rogers GT, Blumberg JB, Au R, DeCarli C, Jacques PF. "Flavonoid Intake and MRI Markers of Brain Health in the Framingham Offspring Cohort." *J Nutr*. Jun 1 2020;150(6):1545-1553. doi:10.1093/jn/nxaa068.

449. Berg S. "What doctors wish patients knew about vitamins and supplements." https://www.ama-assn.org/print/pdf/node/75286. Accessed October 9, 2021.

450. Cohen PA, Avula B, Wang YH, Zakharevich I, Khan I. "Five unapproved drugs found in cognitive enhancement supplements." *Neurol Clin Pract*. 2020.

451. White CM. "Continued Risk of Dietary Supplements Adulterated With Approved and Unapproved Drugs: Assessment of the US Food and Drug Administration's Tainted Supplements Database 2007 Through 2021." *J Clin Pharmacol*. Aug 2022;62(8):928-934. doi:10.1002/jcph.2046.

452. "Apoaequorin (Prevagen) to improve memory." *Med Lett Drugs Ther*. Nov 1 2021;63(1636):175-176.

453. Butler M, Nelson VA, Davila H, et al. "Over-the-Counter Supplement Interventions to Prevent Cognitive Decline, Mild Cognitive Impairment, and Clinical Alzheimer-Type Dementia: A Systematic Review." *Ann Intern Med*. Jan 2 2018;168(1):52-62. doi:10.7326/m17-1530.

454. Vachon-Presseau E, Berger SE, Abdullah TB, et al. "Brain and psychological determinants of placebo pill response in chronic pain patients." *Nat Commun*. Sep 12 2018;9(1):3397. doi:10.1038/s41467-018-05859-1.

455. Beecher HK. "The powerful placebo." *J Am Med Assoc*. Dec 24 1955;159(17):1602-6. doi:10.1001 /jama.1955.02960340022006.

456. Frumkin K. "Behavioral Conditioning, the Placebo Effect, and Emergency Department Pain Management." *J Emerg Med*. Aug 2020;59(2):303-310. doi:10.1016/j .jemermed.2020.04.025.

457. "Lutein + zeaxanthin and omega-3 fatty acids for age-related macular degeneration: the Age-Related Eye Disease Study 2 (AREDS2) randomized clinical trial." *Jama*. May 15 2013;309(19):2005-15. doi:10.1001 /jama.2013.4997.

458. Scaglione F. "How to Choose the Right *Serenoa repens* Extract." *European Urology Supplements*. 2015;14:e1464-e1469.

459. Vela-Navarrete R, Alcaraz A, Rodríguez-Antolín A, et al. "Efficacy and safety of a hexanic extract of Serenoa repens (Permixon(®)) for the treatment of lower urinary tract symptoms associated with benign prostatic hyperplasia (LUTS/BPH): systematic review and meta-analysis of randomised controlled trials and observational studies." *BJU Int*. Dec 2018;122(6):1049-1065. doi:10.1111/bju.14362.

460. Clayson J. "Certain vapes and medicines banned by FDA are still being sold." Here & Now, National Public Radio, November 16, 2022. https://wwwwburorg /hereandnow/2022/11/16/banned-fda-vape-sales.

461. Bredesen DE. "Reversal of cognitive decline: a novel therapeutic program." *Aging.* Sep 2014;6(9):707-17. doi:10.18632/aging.100690.

462. Bredesen DE, Amos EC, Canick J, et al. "Reversal of cognitive decline in Alzheimer's disease." *Aging.* Jun 2016;8(6):1250-8. doi:10.18632/aging.100981.

463. Rao RV, Kumar S, Gregory J, et al. "ReCODE: A Personalized, Targeted, Multi-Factorial Therapeutic Program for Reversal of Cognitive Decline." *Biomedicines.* Sep 29 2021;9(10). doi:10.3390/biomedicines9101348.

464. McEwen SC, Merrill DA, Bramen J, et al. "A systems-biology clinical trial of a personalized multimodal lifestyle intervention for early Alzheimer's disease." *Alzheimers Dement.* 2021;7(1):e12191. doi:10.1002/trc2.12191.

465. Schechter G, Azad GK, Rao R, et al. "A Comprehensive, Multi-Modal Strategy to Mitigate Alzheimer's Disease Risk Factors Improves Aspects of Metabolism and Offsets Cognitive Decline in Individuals with Cognitive Impairment." *J Alzheimers Dis Rep.* Jun 29 2020;4(1):223-230. doi:10.3233/adr-200185.

466. Keine D, Walker JQ, Kennedy BK, Sabbagh MN. "Development, Application, and Results from a Precision-medicine Platform that Personalizes Multi-modal Treatment Plans for Mild Alzheimer's Disease and At-risk Individuals." *Curr Aging Sci.* 2018;11(3):173-181. doi:10.2174/1874609811666181019101430.

467. Daly T, Mastroleo I, Gorski D, Epelbaum S. "The ethics of innovation for Alzheimer's disease: the risk of overstating evidence for metabolic enhancement protocols." *Theoretical Medicine and Bioethics.* 2020/12/01 2020;41(5):223-237. doi:10.1007/s11017-020-09536-7.

468. Helgesson G. "What is a reasonable framework for new non-validated treatments?" *Theor Med Bioeth*. Dec 2020;41(5-6):239-245. doi:10.1007 /s11017-020-09537-6.

469. Mitrečić D, Petrović DJ, Stančin P, et al. "How to face the aging world—lessons from dementia research." *Croat Med J*. Apr 30 2020;61(2):139-146. doi:10.3325 /cmj.2020.61.139.

470. Thomson H. "How flashing lights and pink noise might banish Alzheimer's, improve memory and more." *Nature*. Mar 2018;555(7694):20-22. doi:10.1038 /d41586-018-02391-6.

471. Grover S, Wen W, Viswanathan V, Gill CT, Reinhart RMG. "Long-lasting, dissociable improvements in working memory and long-term memory in older adults with repetitive neuromodulation." *Nat Neurosci*. Sep 2022;25(9):1237-1246. doi:10.1038 /s41593-022-01132-3.

472. Ngo HV, Martinetz T, Born J, Molle M. "Auditory closed-loop stimulation of the sleep slow oscillation enhances memory." *Neuron*. May 8 2013;78(3):545-53. doi:10.1016/j.neuron.2013.03.006.

473. Wilckens KA, Ferrarelli F, Walker MP, Buysse DJ. "Slow-Wave Activity Enhancement to Improve Cognition." *Trends Neurosci*. Jul 2018;41(7):470-482. doi:10.1016/j .tins.2018.03.003.

474. Budson AE, Solomon PR. "Future Treatments of Memory Loss, Alzheimer's Disease, and Dementia." *Memory Loss, Alzheimer's Disease and Dementia*. 3 ed. Elsevier; 2022:237-253:chap 23.

475. Anderson P. Anderson, P. "Low-Intensity Focused Ultrasound Safe, Effective in Mild Alzheimer's Disease."

Medscape. Aug 30, 2021. https://www.medscape.com /viewarticle/957487#vp_2.

476. Islam MR, Valaris S, Young MF, et al. "Exercise hormone irisin is a critical regulator of cognitive function." *Nat Metab*. Aug 2021;3(8):1058-1070. doi:10.1038/s42255-021-00438-z.

477. Shapira R, Gdalyahu A, Gottfried I, et al. "Hyperbaric oxygen therapy alleviates vascular dysfunction and amyloid burden in an Alzheimer's disease mouse model and in elderly patients." *Aging*. Sep 9 2021;13(17):20935-20961. doi:10.18632/aging.203485.

478. Goldsmith HS. "Benefit of omental blood flow in Alzheimer's disease: effect on deteriorating neurons." *J Alzheimers Dis*. 2014;42 Suppl 3:S277-80. doi:10.3233 /JAD-132405.

479. Goldsmith HS. "Omentum transposition for treatment of Alzheimer's disease in China." *Chinese Neurosurgical Journal*. 2016/10/10 2016;2(1):39. doi:10.1186 /s41016-016-0060-5.

480. Boehme M, Guzzetta KE, Bastiaanssen TFS, et al. "Microbiota from young mice counteracts selective age-associated behavioral deficits." *Nature Aging*. Aug 9 2021;1(8):666-676. doi:10.1038/s43587-021-00093-9.

481. Alzheimer's Association. "10 Early Signs and Symptoms of Alzheimer's." https://www.alz.org/alzheimers-dementia/10_signs. Accessed April 21, 2020.

482. AARP. "7 Early Warning Signs of Dementia You Shouldn't Ignore." https://www.aarp.org/caregiving /health/info-2019/dementia-warning-signs.html. Accessed September 3, 2022.

483. Frumkin K. "Toppling Oranges: Death, Disability, Decline, and Readmission of Community-Dwelling Elderly Patients After an Emergency Department Visit."

J Emerg Med. Feb 2020;58(2):339-345. doi:10.1016/j
.jemermed.2019.12.014.

484. Weinstein AM, Gujral S, Butters MA, et al. "Diagnostic
Precision in the Detection of Mild Cognitive
Impairment: A Comparison of Two Approaches." *Am
J Geriatr Psychiatry.* Apr 14 2021;doi:10.1016/j
.jagp.2021.04.004.

485. Beversdorf DQ, Nagaraja HN, Bornstein RA, Scharre
DW. "The Effect of Donepezil on Problem-solving
Ability in Individuals With Amnestic Mild Cognitive
Impairment: A Pilot Study." *Cogn Behav Neurol.*
Sep 2 2021;34(3):182-187. doi:10.1097
/WNN.0000000000000280

486. *Dementia: Ethical Issues.* London: Nuffield Council on
Bioethics, 2009. https://www.nuffieldbioethics.org
/assets/pdfs/Dementia-report-for-web.pdf. Accessed
June 22, 2022.

487. Kolata G. "Alzheimer's Tests Soon May Be Common.
Should You Get One?" *New York Times*, July 28, 2020.
https://www.nytimes.com/2019/12/20/health
/alzheimers-disease-diagnosis.html. Accessed April 30,
2021.

488. Wolk DA, Dickerson BC. "Clinical features and
diagnosis of Alzheimer's disease.," in UpToDate, S.
DeKosky and J.L. Wilterdink, editors. 2022.

489. Stites SD, Karlawish J, Harkins K, Rubright JD,
Wolk D. "Awareness of Mild Cognitive Impairment
and Mild Alzheimer's Disease Dementia Diagnoses
Associated With Lower Self-Ratings of Quality of Life
in Older Adults." *J Gerontol B Psychol Sci Soc Sci.* Oct 1
2017;72(6):974-985. doi:10.1093/geronb/gbx100.

490. Schicktanz S, Schweda M, Ballenger JF, et al. "Before
it is too late: professional responsibilities in late-onset
Alzheimer's research and pre-symptomatic prediction."

Front Hum Neurosci. 2014;8:921. doi:10.3389 /fnhum.2014.00921.

491. Huijbers W, Papp KV, LaPoint M, et al. "Age-Related Increases in Tip-of-the-tongue are Distinct from Decreases in Remembering Names: A Functional MRI Study." *Cereb Cortex.* Sep 1 2017;27(9):4339-4349. doi:10.1093/cercor/bhw234.

492. Shaw Q. "On aphorisms." *Br J Gen Pract.* 2009;59(569):954-955.

493. "Talking to Your Family About an Alzheimer's Diagnosis." Chester County Hospital's *Health e-Living Blog,* April 13, 2022. https://www.chestercountyhospital.org/news /health-eliving-blog/2022/april/talking-to-your-family -about-an-alzheimers-diagnosis. Accessed May 7, 2022.

494. Marcantonio ER. "Delirium in Hospitalized Older Adults." *N Engl J Med.* Oct 12 2017;377(15):1456-1466. doi:10.1056/NEJMcp1605501.

495. Inouye SK. "A practical program for preventing delirium in hospitalized elderly patients." *Cleve Clin J Med.* Nov 2004;71(11):890-6. doi:10.3949/ccjm.71.11.890.

496. Frumkin K. "How to Survive the Emergency Room." *AARP Bulletin.* Apr 2021. p. 30-33.

497. Krumholz HM. "Post-hospital syndrome—an acquired, transient condition of generalized risk." *N Engl J Med.* Jan 10 2013;368(2):100-2. doi:10.1056/NEJMp1212324.

498. Palese A, Gonella S, Moreale R, et al. "Hospital-acquired functional decline in older patients cared for in acute medical wards and predictors: Findings from a multicentre longitudinal study." *Geriatr Nurs.* May-Jun 2016;37(3):192-9. doi:10.1016/j.gerinurse.2016.01.001.

499. Haynesworth A, Gilmer TP, Brennan JJ, et al. "Clinical and financial outcome impacts of comprehensive geriatric assessment in a level 1 geriatric emergency

department." *J Am Geriatr Soc.* Jul 12 2023;doi:10.1111 /jgs.18468.

500. Gallo F, DeLuca V, Prystauka Y, Voits T, Rothman J, Abutalebi J. "Bilingualism and Aging: Implications for (Delaying) Neurocognitive Decline." *Front Hum Neurosci.* 2022;16:819105. doi:10.3389/fnhum.2022.819105.

501. Uncapher MR, Wagner AD. "Minds and brains of media multitaskers: Current findings and future directions." *Proc Natl Acad Sci U S A.* Oct 2 2018;115(40):9889-9896. doi:10.1073/pnas.1611612115.

502. Maxwell CJ, Alkabbani W, Yasar S. "Pioglitazone and Lower Risk of Dementia: Will This Change Practice?" *Neurology.* Apr 25 2023;100(17):803-804. doi:10.1212 /wnl.0000000000207182.

503. Shaw G. "Can Household Chores Be Considered Brain-Boosting Exercise?," in *Brain&Life,* https://www .brainandlife.org/articles/doing-household-chores-may -be-good-for-your-brain#:~:text=The%20new%20 findings%20also%20correlate,by%20balance%20 and%20coordination%20tests. Accessed May 6, 2023. 2023.

504. Alateeq K, Walsh EI, Cherbuin N. "Dietary magnesium intake is related to larger brain volumes and lower white matter lesions with notable sex differences." *Eur J Nutr.* Mar 10 2023;doi:10.1007/s00394-023-03123-x.

505. Yang Z, Wei C, Li X, et al. "Association Between Regular Laxative Use and Incident Dementia in UK Biobank Participants." *Neurology.* 2023;100(16):e1702-e1711. doi:10.1212/wnl.0000000000207081.

506. Kulshreshtha A, Alonso A, McClure LA, Hajjar I, Manly JJ, Judd S. "Association of Stress With Cognitive Function Among Older Black and White US Adults."

JAMA Network Open. 2023;6(3):e231860-e231860. doi:10.1001/jamanetworkopen.2023.1860.

507. Kim KY, Kim EH, Lee M, Ha J, Jung I, Kim E. "Restless leg syndrome and risk of all-cause dementia: a nationwide retrospective cohort study." *Alzheimer's Research & Therapy.* 2023/03/06 2023;15(1):46. doi:10.1186/s13195-023-01191-z.

508. Chacko A, Delbaz A, Walkden H, et al. "Chlamydia pneumoniae can infect the central nervous system via the olfactory and trigeminal nerves and contributes to Alzheimer's disease risk." *Scientific Reports.* 2022/02/17 2022;12(1):2759. doi:10.1038/s41598-022-06749-9.

509. Xiao T, Ghatan S, Mooldijk SS, et al. "Association of Bone Mineral Density and Dementia." *The Rotterdam Study.* 2023;100(20):e2125-e2133. doi:10.1212/wnl.0000000000207220.

510. Laine C, Winker MA. "Identifying Predatory or Pseudo-Journals." World Association of Medical Editors. Feb 15 2017. http://www.wame.org .

511. Morran C. "We Dissected This Fake News Site Linking Denzel, Stephen Hawking To Brain-Boosting Pills." https://www.consumerreports.org/consumerist/ridiculous-fake-news-site-falsely-claims-denzel-washington-stephen-hawking-endorse-brain-boosting-pills/. Accessed June 27, 2020.

512. Cantor NL. "On Avoiding Deep Dementia." *Hastings Cent Rep.* Jul 2018;48(4):15-24. doi:10.1002/hast.865.

513. Cantor NL. My annotated living will. *Law Med Health Care.* Spring-Summer 1990;18(1-2):114-22. doi:10.1111/j.1748-720x.1990.tb01139.x.

514. Sara Davidson: "'Pleasant Dementia' and Inner Peace." *Newsweek*, September 12, 2008. https://wwwnewsweekcom/

sara-davidson-pleasant-dementia-and-inner-peace-88517. Accessed July 24, 2022.

515. Montaruli A, Castelli L, Mulè A, et al. "Biological Rhythm and Chronotype: New Perspectives in Health." *Biomolecules*. Mar 24 2021;11(4). doi:10.3390 /biom11040487.

516. Sessums LL, Zembrzuska H, Jackson JL. "Does this patient have medical decision-making capacity?" *JAMA*. Jul 27 2011;306(4):420-7. doi:10.1001/jama.2011.1023.

517. Leebov W. "'But I meant well!'" *Language of Caring*. 2014;6(63):1-5.

518. Bonnesen JL, Burgess EO. "Senior moments: The acceptability of an ageist phrase." *Journal of Aging Studies*. 2004;18(2):123-142.

519. Alzheimer's Disease International. 2019. "World Alzheimer Report 2019: Attitudes to dementia." London: Alzheimer's Disease International.

520. Yasgur BS. "Age-Related Cognitive Decline Not Inevitable?" Medscape. Apr 6, 2021. https://www .medscape.com/viewarticle/948770. Accessed July 22, 2022.

521. Beker N, Ganz A, Hulsman M, et al. "Association of Cognitive Function Trajectories in Centenarians With Postmortem Neuropathology, Physical Health, and Other Risk Factors for Cognitive Decline." *JAMA Netw Open*. Jan 4 2021;4(1):e2031654. doi:10.1001 /jamanetworkopen.2020.31654.

522. Sommerlad A, Mukadam N. "Evaluating risk of dementia in older people: a pathway to personalized prevention?" *Eur Heart J*. Nov 1 2020;41(41):4034-4036. doi:10.1093/eurheartj/ehaa691.

523. Juul Rasmussen I, Rasmussen KL, Nordestgaard BG, Tybjærg-Hansen A, Frikke-Schmidt R. "Impact of

cardiovascular risk factors and genetics on 10-year absolute risk of dementia: risk charts for targeted prevention." *Eur Heart J.* Nov 1 2020;41(41):4024-4033. doi:10.1093/eurheartj/ehaa695.

524. "Abstract: Symposia, Conferences, Oral communications: 14th Clinical Trials on Alzheimer's Disease (CTAD)" November 9-12, 2021. *J Prev Alzheimers Dis.* 2021;8(S1):S2-s72. doi:10.14283/jpad.2021.57.

525. "Abstract: Posters: 14th Clinical Trials on Alzheimer's Disease (CTAD)" November 9-12, 2021. *J Prev Alzheimers Dis.* 2021;8(S1):S73-s170. doi:10.14283/jpad.2021.58.

526. Hudomiet P, Hurd MD, Rohwedder S. "Trends in inequalities in the prevalence of dementia in the United States." *Proc Natl Acad Sci U S A.* Nov 16 2022;119(46):e2212205119. doi:10.1073/pnas.2212205119.

527. Langa KM, Larson EB, Crimmins EM, et al. "A Comparison of the Prevalence of Dementia in the United States in 2000 and 2012." *JAMA internal medicine.* Jan 1 2017;177(1):51-58. doi:10.1001/jamainternmed.2016.6807.

528. Tom SE, Phadke M, Hubbard RA, Crane PK, Stern Y, Larson EB. "Association of Demographic and Early-Life Socioeconomic Factors by Birth Cohort With Dementia Incidence Among US Adults Born Between 1893 and 1949." *JAMA Netw Open.* Jul 1 2020;3(7):e2011094. doi:10.1001/jamanetworkopen.2020.11094.

529. Harvey PD. "Domains of cognition and their assessment." *Dialogues Clin Neurosci.* Sep 2019;21(3):227-237. doi:10.31887/DCNS.2019.21.3/pharvey.

530. Custodio N, Lira D, Herrera-Perez E, et al. "Memory Alteration Test to Detect Amnestic Mild Cognitive Impairment and Early Alzheimer's Dementia in

Population with Low Educational Level." *Front Aging Neurosci*. 2017;9:278. doi:10.3389/fnagi.2017.00278.

531. Elwyn G, Frosch D, Thomson R, et al. "Shared decision making: a model for clinical practice." *J Gen Intern Med*. Oct 2012;27(10):1361-7. doi:10.1007 /s11606-012-2077-6.

532. Cahill S. "WHO's global action plan on the public health response to dementia: some challenges and opportunities." *Aging Ment Health*. Feb 2020;24(2):197–199. doi:10.1080/13607863.2018.1544213.

533. *A blueprint for dementia research*. Geneva: World Health Organization; 2022.

534. National Academies of Sciences, Engineering, and Medicine 2015. "The Space Science Decadal Surveys: Lessons Learned and Best Practices." Washington, DC: The National Academies Press. https://doi .org/10.17226/21788.

535. National Academies of Sciences, Engineering, and Medicine. In: Schulz R, Eden J, eds. *Families Caring for an Aging America*. 2016.

INDEX

ABOUT THE AUTHOR

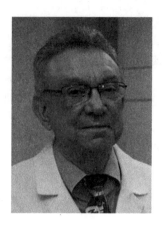

Kenneth Frumkin, PhD, MD, FACEP studied physiological psychology (the interaction of the body's basic biologic and neurologic mechanisms with behavior) in college and graduate school. He earned his master's and PhD degrees from McGill University for his work on the relative contributions of nature and nurture to the ingrained survival mechanism of poison-avoidance in rats.

After two years of research at the US Army's Biomedical Laboratories, mainly studying mechanisms of addiction in animals, he went on to medical school and a residency in emergency medicine. His thirty-six-year medical career was split between community hospital emergency departments and teaching, research, and practice in military academic medical centers.

Board certified in his specialty, Dr. Frumkin is the author of over three dozen peer-reviewed publications and textbook chapters in psychology and medicine. (See References 1-15. A complete list and resume is available at www.linkedin.com/in/KennethFrumkinPhDMD.)

Having retired as a civilian employee of the Department of the Navy in 2017, Dr. Frumkin is currently a volunteer member of the academic faculty at the Emergency Medicine Residency, Naval Medical Center, Portsmouth, Virginia.

Dr. Frumkin writes from the perspective of a practiced author and researcher and, most importantly, as a fellow senior citizen with "skin in the game." He, too, is seeking the answers to nearly every older-person's questions about their fluctuating memories and the possibility of progressive cognitive decline.